The Child in the Centre

Seventy-Five Years
at the
Alberta
Children's Hospital

❖❖❖❖❖❖❖❖❖❖❖

*All the best to
Tom O'Connor*

Arty

Arty Coppes-Zantinga
Ian Mitchell

University of Calgary Press
2500 University Drive N.W.
Calgary, Alberta, Canada T2N 1N4

Canadian Cataloguing in Publication Data
Coppes-Zantinga, Arty, 1958-
  The child in the centre

  ISBN 1-895176-99-9

  1. Alberta Children's Hospital—History. I. Mitchell, Ian,
1943—II. Title.
RJ28.C34C66 1997   362.1'9892'0009712338   C97-910682-6

COMMITTED TO THE DEVELOPMENT OF CULTURE AND THE ARTS

♾ This book is printed on acid-free paper.

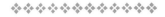

Dedication on plaque commemorating
the opening of the Child Health Centre
September 10, 1981

The Child Health Centre is dedicated
to Alberta's most precious resource
– our children –
Here, care extends to the spirit, as well as to the body;
the prevention of illness
is fundamental; the regard for
the family and the involvement of
the community are foremost.

The text was developed by the staff and
Board of the Alberta Children's Hospital in 1981.

This plaque was recently placed in the Child Space.

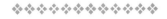

ABBREVIATIONS

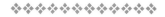

AARN	Alberta Association of Registered Nurses
ACH	Alberta Children's Hospital
ACHF	Alberta Children's Hospital Foundation
AMA	Alberta Medical Association
CHAS	Children's Hospital Aid Society
CHC	Child Health Centre (of Alberta Children's Hospital)
CMA	Canadian Medical Association
CNA	Canadian Nurses Association
CP	Cerebral Palsy
CPR	Canadian Pacific Railway
CPSA	College of Physicians and Surgeons of Alberta
CRHA	Calgary Regional Health Authority
CT	Computed Tomography
DAT	Centre Diagnostic, Assessment and Treatment Centre
ECG	Electrocardiogram
EEG	Electroencephalogram
FRCPC	Fellow of the Royal College of Physicians Canada
GWVA	Great War Veterans' Association
ICU	Intensive Care Unit
LMCC	Licence of the Medical Council of Canada
MRI	Magnetic Resonance Imaging
NWMP	Northwest Mounted Police
NWTMA	Northwest Territories Medical Association
PCDC	Providence Child Development Centre
PICU	Paediatric Intensive Care Unit
PPS	Post-Polio Syndrome
RCPSC	Royal College of Physicians and Surgeons of Canada
RN	Registered Nurse
SAIT	Southern Alberta Institute of Technology
STARS	Shock Trauma Air Rescue Society
UNA	United Nurses of Alberta
VON	Victorian Order of Nurses
YMCA	Young Men's Christian Association
NICU	Neonatal Intensive Care Unit
HR	Health Records
HR	Human Resources

CONTENTS

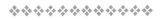

FOREWORD

❖❖❖❖❖❖❖❖❖❖❖❖❖❖

by Grant McEwan

It gives me great pleasure to introduce the history of the seventy-five-year-old Alberta Children's Hospital. In the late 1940s, when I moved to Calgary, I was told that there were two important things in town: the Children's Hospital and the Zoo on St. George's Island! Throughout the years, the great reverence in which the citizens held the Children's Hospital has been very obvious to me. And rightfully so! The Alberta Children's Hospital has gained a special place in the hearts of many, or all, Calgarians because of its unique dedication to our children. I remember visiting the Children's Hospital in the early 1950s and being impressed by the respect for its patients.

Since then, Calgary has grown tremendously, evolving from a small city, where 8th Avenue was still a friendly lane, to a lively and dynamic city with almost 800,000 people. Respect for the Children's Hospital has not been lost. It is true that recent cutbacks have made it harder for institutions such as the Children's Hospital to continue to fulfill their commitment to sick children and their families. Fortunately, Calgarians have remained supportive of its world-class children's hospital.

Let's hope that in this year of celebration, Calgarians will renew their support for their Children's Hospital, and the staff will retain their loyalty to the care of sick children.

Grant McEwan

FOREWORD

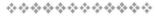

by Dr. Grant Gall

The Alberta Children's Hospital reflects the community in which we live. The Alberta Children's Hospital has been and continues to be an integral part of the community and continues to receive strong public support for its existence and role. Since its inception, the Alberta Children's Hospital has strived to be a Centre of Excellence for the health care of children of Calgary, southern Alberta and Alberta. The hospital, initiated as a facility for the care of chronically ill children, has evolved to a major Centre of Excellence for Child Health Care in Canada. The Alberta Children's Hospital has taken its place as a leading academic tertiary care facility for child health. In these turbulent times of change in health care, it is reassuring and comforting to witness a continued strong relationship between the community and the hospital. The Alberta Children's Hospital has a special place in the hearts of Calgarians and Albertans. This ongoing relationship will ensure that the children of southern Alberta have access to the finest health care in Canada. I congratulate the authors for their efforts in recording the history of the Alberta Children's Hospital. As we move forward we must not lose touch with our past.

A Message from

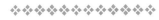

Mayor Al Duerr

O n behalf of City Council and the citizens of Calgary, it gives me great pleasure to acknowledge the history of the Alberta Children's Hospital. The 75th anniversary of this unique organization for children allows us to recognize one of the many ways in which Calgarians have helped children.

In 1922, the Alberta Children's Hospital was in a house on 18th Avenue SW and had very few staff. Since then, there have been two moves and one major expansion, and now we have a comprehensive child health centre with many highly skilled staff. The Children's Hospital, like our city, has had many different leaders and has experienced significant growth. However, the underlying values of the Alberta Children's Hospital have not changed. Children and parents continue to enjoy personal and individual attention. Our citizens share their appreciation of this family-friendly organization with many who come from other parts of Alberta, and indeed some who come from outside the province.

Calgarians are proud of the Alberta Children's Hospital and together we all look forward to the future.

Sincerely,

All Duerr
MAYOR

PREFACE

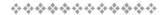

T he idea of recording the history of the Alberta Children's Hospital came after a late evening conversation between the authors, not long after the events of 1994 when the hospital had to fight for its life. We realized that the Alberta Children's Hospital had been in existence since 1922 and would soon have its seventy-fifth anniversary. This was an event that should be commemorated. When we started our exploration, we were helped by records that had already been put together by Dorothy Potts and Audrey Manning.

The high regard in which the hospital is held in the community of Calgary and southern Alberta and the pride of those who work in the hospital became more and more obvious as we explored the history. This high regard and pride are well placed, and we identified many innovative ideas put into practice at the Alberta Children's Hospital over the years.

Our task was to write an accurate and scholarly history that would still be interesting to the general reader, to parents and children who had used the hospital and to hospital staff. We also wanted to convey the warmth and care given in this hospital over the years. Primary sources of information were therefore important and included the *Minutes* of the Alberta Division of The Canadian Red Cross Society, which detailed much of the early material regarding the foundation of the hospital, and the *Minutes* of the Alberta Children's Hospital Foundation, which owned the hospital for a time. The generosity with which individuals and organizations were willing to share their ideas, memories and records with us was impressive. Unfortunately, we were not given access to relevant parts of the *Minutes* of the Foothills Hospital Board or the Alberta Children's Hospital Board, which may have helped us to understand the period 1966-82 better. However, we had considerable first-hand information, access to official reports and press accounts.

We were blessed with wonderfully talented and enthusiastic volunteers who brought energy, enthusiasm and unique skills to the job. Dorothy Potts, a former Director of Nursing and as young as the hospital, not only brought enormous energy, but also endless stories and recollections. Dorothy is a legend in the Alberta Children's Hospital, and the fact that she was associated with us helped open many doors, even to the point where she found furniture for our office. Mona Donckerwolcke did extensive research at the Glenbow and helped classify data and pictures in her meticulous way. Anne Mitchell, who has a background in nursing and library technology, created an archive of hospital records and photographs on the computer and helped identify references and choose pictures for the book. Ralph Hodgins, former Principal of the Dr. Gordon Townsend School, helped in the completion of the history of the Dr. Gordon Townsend School. Inga and Martin Holtz also assisted with various projects.

The process of writing led to many drafts, and the book could not have been produced without the endless patience of Diane Beauvais-Bishop, who not only transformed our untidy script into a new version every time, but also indicated where the text could be improved. Maureen Ranson used great skill and dedication in polishing and improving the text and in ensuring that our message was clearly understood. The authors shared the task of research and writing equally.

This is the story of one community and one institution and attempts to give an overall view of the many changes that have taken place in Canadian society and in health care through the course of this century. The successes and struggles of the Alberta Children's Hospital (ACH) are described in six main parts. Part I is general background information and deals with wider paediatric issues to set the scene. Parts II through VI are chronological. Part VII highlights, the school, volunteers, and support staff, "constants" in the life of ACH. In Part I, the sections dealing with paediatrics and nursing present an overview to help the reader understand professional developments relevant to ACH. We do not claim to have provided detailed histories of these topics. It is unavoidable that these two sections refer to events that are described in detail elsewhere in the book, and we hope the reader is not confused.

While the theme of this book is clear, with its focus on child health in Calgary, the sources available to us varied widely. Until 1952, these were mainly personal accounts. In the second half of the history, there was an abundance of personal memories and official records. This is reflected with greater emphasis on political detail necessary to help the reader evaluate the decisions made in the last three decades.

The hospital has had many names, and we have attempted to use the one appropriate for each stage in the life of the hospital, but occasionally we use the general term "Alberta Children's Hospital." We have chosen traditional spellings for "paediatrics" and "orthopaedics," as these were in use throughout most of the life of the hospital.

We acknowledge gratefully the support of the Alberta Children's Hospital Foundation for funding the early parts of this study and publication costs; the Board of Directors and Administrators of the Alberta Children's

Hospital (before the Board was dissolved in 1995), who encouraged the project; Calgary Regional Health Authority and Child Health Program Administration, especially Senior Operating Officer, Nora Greenley; The University of Calgary, particularly Dr. Grant Gall, Head of the Department of Paediatrics; The University of Calgary Press, which gave us great help throughout the project; and everyone who shared memories with us either through interviews or photographs. The following people were particularly helpful: Becky Ashenhurst, Dr. Philip Barker, Margaret Baxter, Bill Bloss, Jan Bruneau, Dr. Ian Burgess, Grant Christensen, Dr. Margaret Clarke, Lorna Clogg, Margaret Coleman, Dr. Peter Cruse, Dr. Sam Darwish, Phyllis Davis, Linda Dearden, Dr. Taj Jadavji, Reny de Jong, Elizabeth Denham, Judy Duce, Kelly Duregon, Margaret Dykes, Dr. Glen Edwards, Dr. Ehor Gauk, Jim Goodwin, Don Graves, Dr. Lloyd Grisdale, Dr. Robert Haslam, Pauline Height, Jim Herbisson, Dr. Warren Hindle, John Huggett, Bob Innes, Kay Jamieson, Gaye Kavanagh, Janet Ross Kerr, Kim Kerrone, Val Lange, Marie Laroque, Irene Long, Dr. Brian Lowry, Doreen (*née* Christie) Lyall, Audrey Manning, Ken Manning, Eva Marvin, J. Mather, Sandi Miki, Neil Mitchell, Betty Moffat, Dr. Joe Moghadam, Anne Myles, Helen (*née* Christie) MacIntosh, Amanda McCord, Jean McQuilliam, Marie McKay, Cathy McKinnon, Betty McRobbie, Tom O'Connor, Margi Ramsay, Judy Raynor, Juliette Richards, Jean Roberts, Janice Robertson, Christopher Rutty, Dr. Goeff Seagram, Peggy Soutar, Dr. David Stephure, Astrid Storry, Dr. Gordon Townsend, Linda Traquair, Shannon Turnbull, Jean Tyler, Dale Wicki, and Shirley Wormsbecker.

Unless otherwise stated, all photos are from the Alberta Children's Hospital Archives. Judy Pedersen created graphs from data supplied by the authors; Carol Petersen, diagrams of cluster layout; and Jocelyn Skutelnik and Leslie Herchak, the floor plans of the hospital.

Many of those who have played a major role in the hospital are mentioned, but we could not mention everyone by name. This does not mean that their contributions to child care were not important or not valued by us. While the story of the Alberta Children's Hospital is one of success through dedication, patience and perseverance, we might on occasion fall short of describing what this hospital has meant and continues to mean to our community and individual members. If so, the omission is ours.❖

PART ONE

INTRODUCTION

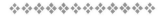

Life in Calgary in the 1920s

The Alberta Children's Hospital officially opened on its first site in 1922 in a world which seems very different from life today. However, we probably have more in common with the citizens of Calgary in 1922 than we have differences. They desired a good life for themselves and their families, wished to have jobs and recreation, pursued education, and had hobbies and sports. There were, of course, differences. The founding of the Province of Alberta (1905) was still a recent memory for many citizens. The whole population had been affected by the recent World War I. Those who had stayed in Alberta during the war saw many changes. In agriculture there was massive wheat production, and the major industries (mining and forestry) had undergone tremendous expansion to meet wartime requirements. Those who went abroad during the war lost many of their comrades. On their return, they found many changes including income tax, daylight saving time and prohibition of alcohol, all introduced as wartime measures. The role of women changed; women had become a major part of the work force and entered political life. Women gained the vote in Alberta in 1916, and a year later, two women (Louise McKinney and Roberta McAdams) were elected to the Provincial Legislature. In Calgary, Annie Gale became the first Alderman in the British Empire in 1918. Women were given the vote in the rest of Canada in 1918.

In 1922, life at home was changing fast. Electricity had reached every city home by 1920 and was spreading to rural areas. Appliances, stoves, toasters, vacuum cleaners and washers were revolutionizing life at home. Outside the home, street lights were bright, visible from as far away as Okotoks (40 km from Calgary). There were movie theatres, and later in the decade, the first movie with sound came to Calgary. Automobiles were becoming more common, and roads were developing, with gas stations sprouting along the highway to meet the needs of travellers on business or vacation. Despite this, rail was still the main mode of transport,

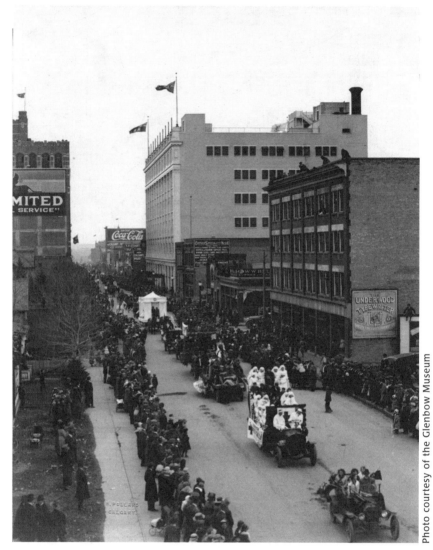

Photo courtesy of the Glenbow Museum

Stampede parade, 1926.

and the extensive network which had sprung up during the war continued
to expand during the 1920s to meet personal and industrial needs.

Western Canada had long cold winters, and so winter sports were very
important in recreation. There was skating on the Elbow River and an
indoor rink (the Crystal Rink) on 7th Avenue SW.

In 1921, the Stampede decided to sponsor the Calgary Winter Carni-
val. Skiers could jump from a specially built steel tower (75') and slope,
and success was ensured by bringing in many tons of snow. There were

eleven thousand spectators. The next year, there was a Chinook, and more snow had to be imported from Lake Louise in railway cars. On the actual day of jumping, disaster struck! An arctic gale ensured that less than one thousand spectators attended.[1]

In summer, there was tennis and football. There was dancing at MacDonald's Dancing Academy on 12th Avenue SW for young people. The more affluent dined at the Palliser. Many left the city on weekends to see the Barnstormers, who were ex-wartime flyers, one of them the famous McCall. They gave demonstrations of flying and took the public for short flights, using the fields of co-operative farmers for takeoff and landing.

The first Exhibition was in 1884, and by 1922 attendance was 97,732.[2] The first Stampede was in 1912, and the second was held in 1919 to celebrate the victory of the allies. Attendance was 57,456.[3] In 1923, the annual Agriculture Exhibition joined the Stampede.[4] The combined event was an instant success. This year also saw the start of the chuckwagon breakfasts. A camp cook who had come on one of the wagons gave in to an impulse, lit a fire, made pancakes and handed them out. Thus a tradition was born.[5]

The national parks were important. Their origin lay in a desire both to preserve natural beauty and to promote tourism. Banff National Park was approved in 1885.[6] By 1922, Banff and Lake Louise were prime tourist destinations for the wealthy of North America and Europe, and the first road to Windermere opened that year.[7] All of the national parks in Canada, including Banff and Jasper national parks, brought $18 million dollars into the country's economy.

Oil had been discovered at Turner Valley (Dingman well) on May 14, 1914, and oil exploration became a major preoccupation. Finding more oil in the succeeding decade led to Imperial Oil building a refinery in 1922. Overall, the oil industry made an enormous difference to the economy of Alberta and is still a major economic force today.

There was a marked increase in economic activity during the war, which continued in the post-war period, although this was not uniform across all sectors of society nor in all industries. For example, the dry weather between 1918 and 1922 posed major problems for farmers in the Prairies. Many new companies were formed in Canada in 1922, such as the Hamilton Tire and Rubber Company Limited, which subsequently became Canadian Tire.

Overall, the population had undergone tremendous change in the previous two hundred years and was still changing. In the late seventeen hundreds and through the eighteen hundreds, there were a few fur traders, but the population of the North West Territories, precursor of Alberta, was overwhelmingly Native people. Tremendous immigration started late in the nineteenth century and intensified in the first decade of the twentieth century. It slowed a little, but did not stop, during the war, so that by the end of the war, Native people were in the minority. In 1921, the population of Alberta was 588,454 and only 2.5 percent were Native people. Not only had many European people come to Alberta, but the Native people had a high death rate associated with unfamiliar diseases, malnutrition and difficulties adjusting to a different way of life. In 1921, the majority of the non-Native population was of British descent, either born in Alberta or recent immigrants, although those born in Alberta were in a minority (33%).[8]

In 1922, the Government of Alberta was led by the United Farmers of Alberta, who had defeated the Liberal government in 1921. The United Farmers formed the Alberta Wheat Pool in 1923, based on the idea of co-operative marketing plans of California growers. This organization is still in existence today, although support from farmers is not uniform.

Albertans voted in 1923 to end Prohibition and started selling liquor in government stores only, controlled by the new Liquor Control Board.

In Alberta, women, who had changed their role during the war, took on new responsibilities in addition to gaining the vote. However in 1922, they were still not "persons" legally and could not sit in the Senate. Five Alberta women (Emily Murphy, Irene Parlby, Louise McKinney, Nellie McClung and Henrietta Edwards) were not daunted by defeat on this issue in the Supreme Court of Canada. They took the case further, and, at that time, there was an appeal to the Privy Council in London. The appeal was upheld in 1929, and thus women were finally declared "persons" and could sit in the Senate. A thirty-two-cent stamp honoring Emily Murphy, the leader, was issued in 1985. The Famous Five Foundation was launched in Calgary in 1996, and one of its aims is to create a permanent memorial in Alberta.[9]

There were major advances in communication in Alberta in 1922. The first commercial broadcast was on CJCA in Edmonton by Mayor D.M. Duggan. Calgary followed quickly with CFAC making its first broadcast the next day. The new CFAC radio station was owned by a newspaper, the *Calgary Herald*. The newspapers themselves contained many sports highlights. For example, the public followed the activities of the Edmonton Commercial Grads closely. This was a girls' basketball team, graduates from McDougall Commercial High School, who won their first Canadian title in 1922. That team had unparalleled success over the next fifteen years, winning many awards. They were invited to play as a demonstration sport in the Olympics in Paris in 1924 and won.

Citizens of Calgary were exposed to news not only from their own province but also the world through newspapers and radio. They read the headlines on Dr. Howard Carter opening Tutankhamen's tomb in Egypt, allowing its fabulous treasures to be seen in 1922. They also read about the Indian patriot Ghandi, sentenced to six years imprisonment in March

1922. At that time the role he would play in the independence of India could not be foreseen nor would his future impact as a role model in the use of non-violence be understood.

The media added a new publication with the first issue of Reader's Digest in February 1922. Also on a worldwide level, many of the features of art that are now considered classical were just developing. For example, Salvador Dali was in the forefront of the surrealist movement, as was Pablo Picasso. Sculptor Henry Moore was pre-eminent, and many other art styles, such as the Dutch group "The Style," influenced architecture throughout the 1920s and 1930s.

The status of Canada itself changed. Canada had entered the war automatically as a member of the British Empire, but emerged, at the end of the war, a mature nation. Canada signed the covenant of the League of Nations as one of its founding members.

Health care was also an issue for the public. There was extreme awareness of the need for public health, which was dramatically emphasized by the influenza epidemic of 1919. Soldiers returning from World War I brought this viral infection from Europe to Canada. Before the epidemic had run its course, more than four thousand people had died in Alberta (out of a population of less than 600,000). More people died from influenza after the war than had died as a direct result of the fighting.

Commenting on another health-care problem, which is still present today, the Deputy Minister of Health said "... drug addiction is seen as a growing problem in Canada. There are between 12,000 and 15,000 drug addicts in Canada. It is one of the most critical problems the Department of Health faces nowadays."[10]

The importance of paediatric health care was recognized by the foundation of the Canadian Society for the Study of Diseases of Children in 1922. The name "Canadian Paediatric Society" was proposed in 1922, but was voted down because it was similar to the name used south of the border – American Pediatric Society. In 1951, the Society changed its name to the Canadian Paediatric Society[11], and it has had a leadership role in child health care in Canada from 1922 to the present.

An event of worldwide significance took place in Canada and had particular relevance for child health: the discovery of insulin in 1922. The research team consisted of Dr. Frederick Banting, Dr. Charles Best, Dr. J.J.R. MacLeod and Dr. J.B. Collip. Banting and MacLeod were awarded the Nobel Prize[12] for medicine and physiology in 1923.[13] Insulin, a hormone produced by the pancreas, is important in reducing sugar levels in the body and transforming sugar into energy. This discovery gave hope to people with diabetes mellitus.

Before insulin was available through mass production, the diagnosis of diabetes mellitus in children or adults was a death sentence. A severely restricted carbohydrate diet might prolong the life of the sufferer a little but did not prevent incredible weight loss. During the process of wasting away and dying, people with diabetes had little energy to enjoy life. Diabetes affects 120 million people worldwide. Insulin is still unavailable in many parts of the world. In Africa, for example, a single vial can cost $22, the equivalent of a month's salary.

Dr. James Bertram Collip, whose main role on the research team was to make sure that insulin could be produced and used in patients, was an Albertan. He received his PhD from the University of Toronto and returned to a faculty position at the University of Alberta, but was on sabbatical at the University of Toronto at the time of the study. Dr. J.J.R. MacLeod invited him to join the team. Collip's brilliance as a biochemist[14] enabled him to concentrate pancreatic extracts and develop a form of insulin that could be used in treatment. This scientist was later responsible for the discovery of other significant hormones such as ACTH.

In 1922 , there were a number of minor events, some of which changed the lives of many. It is unlikely that, in 1922, the citizens of Calgary anticipated the tremendous growth of the Alberta Children's Hospital.❖

References

1. Dempsey, Hugh A. *Calgary: The Spirit of the West*. Fifth House, [Calgary] Saksatoon, Glenbow, 1994, pp. 56-60.
2. Gray, James H. *A Brand of its Own: The 100-Year History of the Calgary Exhibition and Stampede*. Western Producer Prairie Books, Saskatoon, 1985, p. 185.
3. Ibid., p. 53.
4. Ibid., p. 58.
5. Ibid., p. 65.
6. Leighton, D., ed. "Banff is where it all began." "Canadian Geographic" (Feb.-March 1985): 8-15.
7. Dempsey, Hugh A. *Calgary: The Spirit of the West*. p. 116.
8. Palmer, H., and T. Palmer, eds. *Peoples of Alberta*. Western Producer Prairie Books, Saskatoon, 1988, pX and XI, 1988.
9. *The Calgary Herald*, October 9, 1996, p. B4.
10. Abbott, Elizabeth, ed.-in-chief. *The Chronicles of Canada*. Chronicles Publications, Montreal, 1990.
11. McKendry, J.B.J., and J.D. Bailey, eds. *Paediatrics in Canada*. Canadian Paediatric Society, Ottawa, 1990, p. 253
12. Nobel prizes were instituted in 1901. Alfred Nobel was a Swedish chemist and inventor, who made a fortune from his most important invention, dynamite. The prizes designated in Nobel's will are for physics, chemistry, physiology or medicine, literature and peace.
13. Bliss, Michael. "J.J.R. MacLeod and the Discovery of Insulin." *Quarterly Journal of Experimental Physiology*, 74 (1989): 87-96.
14. *Canadian Medical Association Journal*, 156 (1997):12-13.

Further reading

Corbet, E.A., and A.W. Rasporich, eds. *Winter Sports in the West*. Historical Society of Alberta, Calgary, 1990.
Hamilton, J. *Our Alberta Heritage*. Calgary Power Ltd., Calgary, June 1977.

Lower, J.A. *Western Canada: An Outline History*. Douglas & McIntyre, Vancouver, 1983.

MacGregor, J.G. *A History of Alberta*. Hurtig, Edmonton, 1981.

McEwan, J.W.G., and M. Foran. *A Short History of Western Canada*. McGraw-Hill Ryerson, Toronto, 1968.

Myers, B.S., and T. Copplestone, eds. *The History of Art*. Viscount Books, Twickenham, England, 1985.

Palmer, H. *Alberta: A New History*. Hurtig, Edmonton, 1990.

Sparks, Susie, ed. *Calgary: A Living Heritage*. 2nd ed. Junior League of Calgary, 1996.

The Spirit of Alberta. Alberta Heritage Foundation, 1979.

Stenson, F. *The Story of Calgary*. Fifth House, Saskatoon, 1994.

Health Care in the 1920s

Today, in the Western world, we expect our children to be healthy. We expect them to be perfect at birth. If there is any problem, we assume it can be corrected. We expect our children to recover rapidly and completely from illnesses. We use skilled physicians. We access hospital care from time to time and expect miracles from modern technology. We know and appreciate that many health-care professionals are involved in delivering these "miracles" to us. In fact, this picture is not far from reality! Nevertheless, it is not reality for all children. Children continue to have congenital abnormalities and continue to develop illnesses. Some of these abnormalities and illnesses are not amenable to treatment, and some can only be partially corrected.

Shifting our focus from the Western world to underdeveloped countries, the situation is not the same. Television, radio, newspapers and magazines inform us all that disease and death in childhood are common. Statistics tell us that many children do not survive the first year and, of those who do, many do not survive childhood. Common infectious disorders are rampant, and nutritional problems are everywhere. It is uncomfortable to look at international statistics. Every year, the World Health Organization publishes the mortality rate of children under five and the mortality rate of children under one (infants), by country.[1] These are given as rates per 1,000 births to allow comparison between different countries. Canada has one of the lowest rates, and Finland is the lowest. Canada's under-five mortality rate in 1993 was 8/1,000 births, and the under-one (infant) mortality rate was 7/1,000 births. This is a remarkable drop from 1921, when the infant mortality rate in Canada was approximately 100/1,000 live births.[2] This means that ten percent of all babies died in the first year of life, which is similar to the current rate in countries such as Kenya and Indonesia and only slightly less than India. Thus, in some ways, Calgary in 1922 resembled the underdeveloped countries of 1997.

In 1922 in Calgary, parents nursed their children through illnesses, no matter how severe, at home. Recovery could take a long time and did not always occur. Indeed most of the deaths were caused by common infectious illnesses that are no longer seen today and, if they still occur are readily treated. Today only two percent of all deaths at any age are preschool children, whereas in 1922, about 33 percent of all deaths were preschool children. There was an awareness and acceptance of the reality of childhood illness and death in all neighborhoods and all walks of life.

Few drugs were effective, surgery was limited, anaesthesia was poorly understood, preventive measures were uncommon, and diagnostic tests were unusual. There were no antibiotics, and indeed the first effective drugs against infection were the sulfonamides introduced in the 1930s. Surgery had made great strides in the late part of the nineteenth century and the early part of the twentieth century, though surgery for children was still not fully recognized as a specialty. Developments in anaesthesia in the nineteenth century were extremely important in allowing more extensive surgery, but anaesthesia still remained primitive, by our standards. Blood transfusions were not available even for major trauma, and saline solutions were not given intravenously. Smallpox vaccination was recognized as successful, but most other immunizations we take for granted were not in routine use. X-rays had been introduced for diagnosis at the end of the nineteenth century. The full potential of X-rays, and indeed their danger, was not fully understood in 1922.

Yet there were many positive areas in the development of medicine. For example, orthopaedics had become established and new treatments proposed. Specific training was available for those working in this area. This is particularly relevant since the Alberta Children's Hospital started mainly as an orthopaedic hospital.

In 1922, some of the common orthopaedic disorders arose as the aftermath of infections, others were congenital anomalies. The infections included tuberculosis and osteomyelitis (bone infection), both leading to partial recovery at best. Some of the congenital anomalies that were treated at that time included club foot, congenital dislocation of the hip and orthopaedic problems related to cerebral palsy. Some disorders such as Legg-Perthes' disease and scoliosis could not be classified easily.

Tuberculosis has been a scourge for thousands of years and has even been recognized in ancient Egypt[3] and among "Pre-Columbian Indians."[4] Robert Koch (1843-1910) made numerous discoveries in microbiology while maintaining a country practice far from a university. He was the first to prove that an infection may be caused by a specific micro-organism. Later he moved from his country practice to a prestigious Chair at the University of Berlin and was awarded the 1905 Nobel prize for medicine. His discovery led to a remarkable increase in medicine's understanding of tuberculosis. Tuberculosis itself may affect the lungs, brain, kidney, bones, joints and other parts of the body. It moves from one body system to another in a fairly predictable manner, and the "timetable" of tuberculosis was understood to some extent by 1922. In children, primary infection with tuberculosis affected the lungs, but most children went on to recover spontaneously. In a few children, there was rapid spread of the illness throughout the lungs or the brain, leading to death. Many other children had apparent recovery, but the organism settled in the bones or kidneys, and some years after the acute infection the disease of these organs became obvious.

The general care of the child with tuberculosis was important, particularly nutrition, with the aim of improving the body's general resistance. The germ itself could be killed by ultraviolet rays, and perhaps because of this, or some other reason, direct exposure of the child to sunlight (heliotherapy) was proposed for treatment. This was pioneered in Switzerland and subsequently spread to North America, where children were tanned as part of their treatment. Sunlight was thought to destroy bacteria through a photochemical reaction and lead to systematic improvement in calcium and phosphorus metabolism, as well as improve the appetite and allow the patient to sleep more soundly.[5] We now know that sunlight leads to the formation of Vitamin D in the skin.

In bone and joint tuberculosis, in general, there was a good prospect for recovery if deformities could be avoided. For example, when children were unable to bear their own weight, there were various devices to help the immobilization.

Tuberculosis of the spine is one specific form of bone tuberculosis with many names, such as Pott's disease, spondylitis or Hunchback. In this disease, the vertebrae are destroyed by the disease, and as an individual vertebra crumbles, the vertebrae above and below are therefore at a sharp angle. The Bradford frame, one of many devices to immobilize children, was important in encouraging rest. Despite this severe disease of the spine, some patients could walk provided they had support for the body. For this purpose, the specific support used was called a Paris jacket. Bandages were dipped in wet plaster of Paris and rolled evenly around the body. When the plaster was set, the spine was immobilized. Plaster of Paris was first described by a Flemish army surgeon (Mathijsen, A.) in 1854 and rapidly gained acceptance. Solid and crystalline gypsum is pulverized and ignited at 120°C at which it loses seventy-five percent of its water. The fine white powder that is left is called Plaster of Paris. When water is added, the reaction is reversed, gypsum reforms and can be moulded to hold human limbs in the chosen position.

Osteomyelitis is an infectious disease that often requires long-term treatment. In osteomyelitis, there is direct infection of the bone, and we now know that the organism causing this is almost always *Staphylococcus aureus*. In some children, the illness may be very acute. More commonly, an abscess develops in the bone, then ruptures, and pus is released. New bone is formed at the site of the infection, and the old bone dies and is extruded from the body. Surgery played an important role in osteomyelitis. For example, in the acute phase of the illness, the affected end of the bone would often be opened to allow the pus to drain and, in many children, this was sufficient for a complete recovery. Other children had prolonged discharge of pus from the joint. These children had a different experience; they might have to be in hospital with a leg immobilized for many years and suffered leg length discrepancies and angular deformities as well as stiffened joints.

Orthopaedic treatment was also used in congenital anomalies. There may have been little understanding of the origin of the anomalies, but the impact they had on children was well understood. Club foot was one

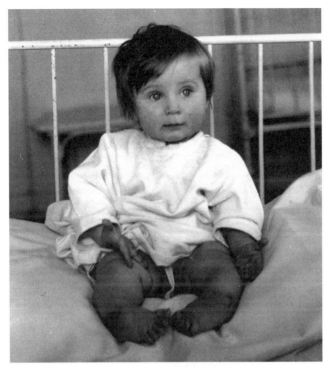

Child with club feet before treatment.

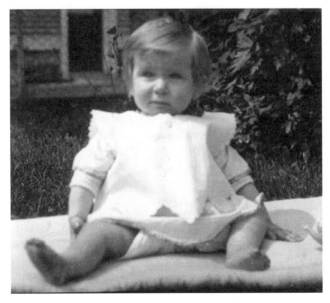

Same child after treatment.

such abnormality and has been recognized throughout history. Club foot can also be an acquired abnormality, after polio, for example. The technical term "equinovarus," comes from the Latin word *equinus* (meaning "horse"), indicating the marked downward direction of the toes, and the Latin word *varus,* which means "crooked."

Treatment for club foot in the 1920s and 1930s started shortly after birth. The feet were wrapped in cotton, and a splint applied on the inner side of the foot pressed the toes outward. Such casts were placed repetitively. Orthopaedic nurses were highly skilled in the splinting of the feet, and they taught their splinting skills to the mothers, who were able to do the manipulation required over an extended period of time. Despite the availability and desirability of treatment after birth, children were usually much older when they were seen. In such children, surgery was required to partially correct the abnormality. Some of these children required braces, which required frequent adjustment by specialized orthopaedic nurses.

Even today, there is confusion about the causes and treatment of club foot. Some children with club foot have muscular or nervous system disease, but, in most children, club foot appears as an isolated congenital anomaly which occurs spontaneously or is inherited. It is still desirable for treatment to start as soon as possible. Plaster is used, or specially constructed boots, but a number of children still require corrective surgery when they have an incomplete result of early casting or splinting treatment.

Congenital dislocation of the hips was rarely diagnosed at birth in the 1920s. Rather, the first sign was an abnormal gait as the child learned to walk, which led to a physician visit and diagnosis. These toddlers required extensive manipulation and often surgery, with convalescence lasting up to eighteen months. Manipulation involved anaesthetizing the child, forcing the leg into the hip socket and then applying a plaster which was left in place for three to six months. In other children, surgery was required. The joint was opened under anaesthesia, the socket examined and the tissues restored as far as possible to normal. The hip bone was then replaced into the socket. Again, plaster was applied to maintain the joint. At the time, it was thought that the results were good, but the best results came when congenital hip displacement was recognized early.

At the present time, all newborn infants are examined immediately after birth or whenever there is any contact with a physician in the first few months of life. If there is any suspicion of hip displacement after this examination, an expert orthopaedic opinion is obtained. If dislocation of the hip is confirmed, splints are applied with an almost uniformly excellent outcome.

Scoliosis is a twisting of the spine and is still not fully understood. It may be seen in young children, but is more commonly seen in teenagers. In 1922, it was thought to be the result of faulty posture or poor diet.

Those with severe scoliosis requiring treatment were stretched. The patient lay on a frame with a pulley at the end, and the spine was pulled straight. This treatment recalls the story of Procrustes in Greek mythology. Procrustes, a giant also known as Polypemon, had one size of bed and insisted his guests fit it exactly. If they were too long for the bed, he cut off whatever part of the body overlapped the edge. If the bed was too long for the guest, he stretched them until they fit. The hero Theseus made Procrustes undergo his own treatment.[6] In the 1920s, if stretching did not work, or the curvature was severe, surgery was followed by bed rest for three months, then several months of mild activity with a brace or plaster jacket. Again authors of the time thought that the outcome was positive with complete cure of mild cases and improvement in more severe cases. Today, scoliosis is commonly seen in children with no other abnormality and in children with neuromuscular disease for whom treatment often involves surgery and requires extensive follow-up. In the group of children with no other abnormality, treatment may be attempted by bracing. A small proportion of patients require corrective surgery. Due to improved spinal fixation devices, prolonged immobilization or body casting is no longer required.

Cerebral palsy remains a complicated illness, that even now is understood incompletely. One subset of the disease is called Little's disease. W.J. Little was born in 1810 and qualified as a physician in 1832. He himself had a club foot secondary to poliomyelitis when he was two years old. Little's disease involves spasticity or stiffening of the muscles of the legs. This is often identified during the first year or in the second year of life. Many different procedures are involved in treatment. These vary from simple stretching of the contracted muscles to invasive surgery. Here the nerve supply to the muscle might be cut, and a contracted spastic muscle will then relax. Many other operations were developed throughout the 1920s and 1930s, but none were any more than partially successful.

Legg-Perthes is an obscure disease which affects children mainly between the ages of three and ten years. This disease was first described by G.C. Perthes (1869-1927), but there are a number of other names such as *coxa plana* and *osteochondritis deformans*. In this disease of the hip bone, there is a loss of the blood supply to part of the head of the femur, because of inflammation or trauma. The children have hip pain and often limp. Physicians find that hip movement is limited. Diagnosis is made by X-ray, which can be used to classify a child's disease in one of several different stages. Full recovery usually occurs in children less than five years of age. In children six years of age and older, the hip may be left with some stiffness. Treatment has varied over the years from rest alone to invasive surgery. Present-day treatment requires short-term rest and traction to reduce inflammation around the hip joint. Surgery is still required today but in a few cases only.

The professions of orthopaedic surgery and orthopaedic nursing developed rapidly even though the conditions treated were not always fully understood. However, the details of treatment were important. Surgeons used manipulation with and without anaesthesia, sequential splinting and surgery, directly exposing bones and joints. Orthopaedic nurses developed specific skills in manipulation and applying braces. Of great importance was the role of nurses in instructing mothers how to carry out treatment at home. Encouraging and teaching parents to look after their own child is continued today by nurses at the Alberta Children's Hospital.

The word orthopaedic itself is interesting. This specialty now deals with patients of all ages, but the word was originally coined by a Parisian surgeon in the seventeenth century (Nicholas André, 1658–1742), and the derivation of orthopaedics from the Greek means "straight child."[7] Dealing with crippled children was always an essential part of the specialty of orthopaedic medicine and orthopaedic surgery. There were certainly developments in orthopaedic medicine and surgery throughout the nineteenth century, and the specialty was well established by the end of that century. In the U.S.A., a number of centres devoted to orthopaedic problems in children developed, and there was a Professor of Orthopaedic Surgery at Bellevue Medical College as early as 1861.[8] Indeed by then, there were a number of hospitals devoted solely to orthopaedics in Great Britain, the first founded in 1838. However, in the late nineteenth century, much of what is now considered orthopaedic care was carried on outside these hospitals by "bone setters." They were knowledgeable and skilled but did not have a formal medical qualification. Bone setters served an apprenticeship, and often there was a family tradition in bone setting which continued for many generations. The pre-eminent bone setters came from the Thomas and Jones families.[9] These families co-operated with one another and even intermarried. Robert Jones was well known in the early part of the twentieth century, but his work had only limited acceptance. This changed dramatically during World War I. War injuries left many soldiers crippled. Orthopaedic treatment had been successful in reducing the number of permanent disabilities resulting from wartime injuries. Jones was a leader in devising treatments and developing a network of hospitals. By the end of the war, there were fifteen orthopaedic centres in Great Britain. Many surgeons came from North America to work with Jones to develop new surgical techniques, at the centres he developed.[10] R.B. Deane was an established surgeon in Calgary who went to England in 1919 (at age 49) for further training. On his return in 1921, he set up practice as the first orthopaedic surgeon in Calgary.[11]

The orthopaedic nurse is described in the book *Crippled Children* by Earl McBride. His description makes it difficult to distinguish an orthopaedic nurse from a saint!

Her care must be minute, definite and perfect in even the smallest item. She must be kind and considerate always. She must be firm in maintaining the exact condition of the appliances being used. Although firm with the patient, she must be gentle, quiet, and soothing, she must continue her efforts on behalf of the patient, regardless of discouragement and apparent non-cooperation of patients and or family. She must have soft, firm flexible fingers and hands that yet are strong and gentle. She must have the sixth sense, acquired by developing qualities of observation and exact technical knowledge of the work, coupled with a true love of this type of nursing. She must overcome everything with patience.[12]

Orthopaedic nurses came from the ranks of general nurses, and it was thought essential that these nurses have good general nursing training, then develop the required orthopaedic skills to a high degree. There was an orthopaedic attitude toward time, patience and respect for accuracy. This so-called orthopaedic attitude related to the after-care required. Surgery might take a few minutes, or a long operation might take two to three hours. However after-care continued for weeks, months and years. Small problems overlooked during this period may, in the long run, lead to a poor outcome and thus major disappointment.

Another profession that developed was the brace maker. Braces are extremely important in orthopaedics and in the treatment of crippled children. The surgeon designed a brace to correct deformity, support limbs or maintain a certain position while healing. The brace maker then made the brace and ensured that it fit the child. Brace makers worked with many different materials, and all braces had to be strong and durable. The joints in particular had to stand up to a great deal of wear.

The psychosocial health of the child requiring long-term treatment was recognized. Children might be in hospital for years, and it was important that they be given some tasks to do that were meaningful. They should be treated, as far as possible, like other children. Attitudes of self-pity were discouraged, and the children were helped to overcome their disabilities by themselves.

A new profession used physical therapy or physiotherapy. As the name indicates, physical agents – light, electricity and water – were used. These physical agents were mainly used to relieve pain, soothe inflammation and stimulate circulation. It was also thought that the treatment might destroy germs. The physical therapy technician required special study in order to understand the physiological effects and limitations of the various forms of electrical modalities and mechanical procedures. Hydrotherapy was widely used as the most practical way of applying heat or cold, using water. There was also another treatment involving water called hydrogymnastics, which originated in an orthopaedic hospital in Los Angeles. The child exercised in warm water, and the principle behind the treatment was the buoyancy of the water used in re-educating body parts. Orthopaedic nurses also needed to be proficient in the use of all of these different physiotherapy treatments, capable of recognizing patients' reactions and symptoms while carrying out the instructed treatment.

The Children's Hospital in Calgary was part of a development in the Western world over the previous two centuries. The first children's hospitals in the modern era were developed to deal with problems of poverty, child abandonment and early parental death, and physicians were not involved to any great extent. One of the early examples was the Foundling Hospital (for children who had been abandoned), which developed due to the energy and drive of a merchant, Thomas Coram, who became rich in the U.S.A. and, on his return to England, was appalled at the distress he saw among children. The first children were admitted in 1741. A similar development took place in Paris later that century, just before the Revolution, but the foundling hospital did not last.[13] However, problems of disease and excessively high mortality in infants were recognized early, with the Hôpital des enfants malades founded in Paris in 1802.[14] Other European cities developed children's hospitals; among the pioneers were: St. Nikolaus Children's Hospital (St. Petersburg, 1824), Vienna (1837),[15] Great Ormond Street (London, 1852).[16] The first American children's hospital was in Philadelphia (1855).[17] Although disease and death were more prevalent in infants than any other age, most of these hospitals did not admit children under two because of a concern that separation from their mother would make death inevitable.

The same trends were seen in Canada. The first hospital was established in the late 1700s in Quebec City for foundlings, and its function was closer to a children's home today. A similar home was developed in Montreal for Protestant orphans.[18] Some of these homes changed gradually into hospitals dealing with disease, but still dealing with the children of the poor since most well-off parents would have their children cared for at home. The first formal children's hospital in Canada, the Hospital for Sick Children in Toronto, was founded in 1875 by a group of determined women.[19] Despite the altruistic motives in attempting to improve conditions for children of the poor who were sick,[20] many of the children admitted died, and among infants the mortality rate was particularly high. This was true of all children's hospitals of the time.

By 1922, Canada had a number of children's hospitals in addition to the Hospital for Sick Children in Toronto. While each was rooted in local altruism and philanthropy, all functioned in different ways and dealt with different aspects of childhood disease. They were: the Children's Memorial Hospital in Montreal, forerunner of the Montreal Children's Hospital (1903), the Children's Hospital in Winnipeg (1909), Ste-Justine Hospital in Montreal (1907), the Children's Hospital in Halifax (1910), the War Memorial Children's Hospital in London, Ontario (1922).

In each of these Canadian cities, enthusiastic volunteers developed what seemed to be appropriate facilities for their city. In Calgary, the Alberta Children's Hospital was designed for children requiring long-term care and orthopaedic treatment. It did not compete with children's units in the General and Holy Cross hospitals which dealt with acute illness. It was about sixty years later that the Alberta Children's Hospital admitted children with both acute and chronic illness.❖

References

1. *The State of the World's Children 1995*. Oxford University Press, 1995.
2. *Selected Infant Mortality and Related Statistics, Canada 1921-1990*. Statistics Canada, 82–549.
3. Stetter, Cornelius, ed. *The Secret Medicine of the Pharaohs: Ancient Egyptian Healing*. Edition Q, Chicago, 1993, p. 70. "In the Egyptian museum in Cairo, there is a statue of a man, about 20 cm high, with a short hump. Scientists have taken this as an indication that bone tuberculosis was present in ancient Egypt."
4. Ackerknecht, Erwin H. *A Short History of Medicine*. Rev. ed. Johns Hopkins University Press, Baltimore, 1982, p. 7.
5. McBride, Earl. *Crippled Children*. Henry Kimpton, London, 1937, pp. 119-224.
6. *New Larousse Encyclopedia of Mythology*. Hamlyn, London, 1959, p. 76.
7. André , N. "L'orthopédie ou l'art de prévenir et de corriger dans les enfants, les difformités du corps." Paris, 1742. In Daniel de Moulin, *A History of Surgery with Emphasis on the Netherlands*. Martinus Nijhoff, Dortrecht, 1988.
8. Siffert, Robert S. "Children's Orthopedic Surgery in the United States: Historical Trends." *Clinical Orthopedics*, 1966 (44): 89-97.
9. Cartwright, F.F. *The Development of Modern Surgery*. Arthur Bokor, London, 1967.
10. Gallie, W.E. "Fifty Years of Orthopedic Surgery." *Medical Clinics of North America*, July 1957: 1101-1109.
11. Edwards, Glen, and D. Harkness. *Life Near the Bone*. Ronalds Printing, Calgary, May 1991, pp. 164-165.
12. McBride, Earl. *Crippled Children*. p. 22.
13. Seidles, E. *An Historical Survey of Children's Hospitals: The Hospital in History*. Ed. Lindsay Granshaw and Roy Porter. Routledge, London , 1989, pp. 101-197.
14. Tixier, Leon. "L'Hôpital des enfants malades," *Cerebral Palsy Bulletin*, 1961, 3(1): 70, Paris.
15. Skopec, M. "Osterreichs erstes Kinderspital," *Clinicum*, (December 1994): 18-19.
16. Wilson, C. "Reports of Continental Childrens' [sic] Hospitals," *Edinburgh Medical Journal*, March 1858.
17. Stokes, Joseph, Jr. "The Children's Hospital of Philadelphia – 100 Years." *Pediatrics*, 16 (1955): 683-687.
18. McKendry, J.B.J., and J.D. Bailey. *Paediatrics in Canada*. Canadian Paediatric Society, Ottawa, 1990, p. 1–3.
19. Braithwaite, M. *Sick Kids: The Story of the Hospital for Sick Children in Toronto*. McClelland & Stewart, Toronto, 1974.
20. Haffey, H. "6 Cots and a Prayer," *The York Pioneer*, 1975, pp. 15-25.

Further reading

Adams, J. C. *Outline of Orthopaedics*, 8th ed. T & A Constable Ltd., Edinburgh, 1976.

Conrad, L., M. Neve, V. Nutton, R. Porter and A. Wear. *The Western Medical Tradition: 800 BC to AD 1800*. Cambridge University Press, 1995.

Granshaw, L., and R. Poter, eds. *The Hospital in History*. Routledge, London, 1989.

Kelland, D. *The Dr. Charles A. Janeway Child Health Centre: A Special Place*. The Children's Hospital Corporation. Robinson Blackmore Printing, St. John's, August 1991.

Klassen, H. "In Search of Neglected and Delinquent Children: The Calgary Children's Aid Society." In *Town and City*, ed. Alan F.J. Artibise, Canadian Plains Research Centre, University of Regina, Regina, 1981.

Medovy, H. *A Vision Fulfilled: History of the Children's Hospital of Winnipeg*, Winnipeg, Peguis, 1979.

Scriver, J.B. *The Montreal Children's Hospital*. McGill-Queen's University Press, 1979.

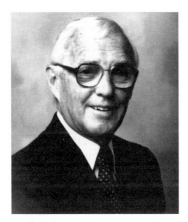

Dr. R.G. (Gordon) Townsend

D r. Townsend was a pioneer in orthopaedics. He was born in 1903 in Woodstock, New Brunswick, trained at McGill and took post-graduate training in Ann Arbor, Michigan, and orthopaedic training abroad.

He came to Calgary in 1939 to assist Dr. Deane, who was still the only orthopaedist in southern Alberta, and succeeded Dr. Deane as Surgeon in Chief. He was responsible for many initiatives in Calgary and Alberta, and the progress of orthopaedics in Alberta and the Alberta Children's Hospital is inseparably linked with his vision.

One major development was the establishment of orthopaedic staff rounds where cases were discussed and treatment programs prepared. He was a co-founder of the Alberta Orthopaedic Society in 1948, although there had been informal regular contacts between established orthopaedic surgeons before this time.

He supported Dr. Glen Edwards in 1960 in starting a residency program with residents rotating from Saskatchewan and Edmonton.

Dr. Townsend continued to serve the hospital long after his retirement, on the Alberta Children's Hospital Foundation Board and as Chair of its Medical Committee. He was actively involved in the Easter Seal Campaign. When there was a competition to name the school in the late 1970s, his contributions were acknowledged by popular acclaim, and Dr. Gordon Townsend graciously lent his name to the school.

He was not only active in the ACH, but also served on numerous local and provincial organizations and in 1966 was president of the Canadian Orthopaedic Society. To commemorate his many activities, the annual R.G. Townsend Lecture is supported by the Calgary Orthopaedic Society and the Alberta Children's Hospital Foundation. This lecture is given by an invited guest speaker in the field of paediatric orthopaedics.

Dramatic Impact of Polio

Polio epidemics from the late 1920s onward, but especially in the early fifties, had a major impact not only on those affected and on the public, but on all hospitals in the Western world. This was particularly true in Calgary, and this one disease had significant influence on the Alberta Children's Hospital and its development. The epidemics led to a purpose-built hospital and to new ways of caring for patients. The end of the epidemic led to a re-evaluation of the hospital's role and the evolution of a broad-based children's hospital rather than solely an orthopaedic centre.

The word "polio" was guaranteed to cast dread into the hearts of parents in the first half of the twentieth century. Now, with the virtual disappearance of polio in North America, it is difficult to fully understand the depth of despair that a polio diagnosis could bring to a family. Perhaps the despair would be closest to the despair felt today by those diagnosed with cancer or AIDS in the Western world. However, polio is still a problem in many parts of the world. In May 1988, representatives of 166 nations meeting at the World Health Assembly in Geneva made the decision to attempt to eradicate polio by the year 2000. This disease still affects many in developing countries, with paralysis occurring in 250,000 children every year, and 23,000 dying. The global elimination of polio is feasible but will require ninety percent immunization rates among children under one year of age for some years, even after no polio cases are reported. The immunization rate reported in the Third World was fifty-five percent in 1989.[1] In 1995, half the world's children under five, 300 million, were immunized during mass campaigns against polio. It is likely that polio will soon be eradicated.[2]

One of the synonyms for polio is "infantile paralysis," a name which describes the most frightening symptom – paralysis – but also gives some indication of the age affected. Although the word infantile is used, this is not a disease of infants in the strict medical sense (i.e., under one year of age), but polio does have a predilection for young people. In fact, infants are relatively resistant to the paralytic effects of the virus. In the early part of the century, with overcrowding and poor hygiene, almost all infants were infected with the polio virus but had a mild infection which conferred long-lasting immunity. Later in the twentieth century, with improvements in hygiene, infants escaped the infection, and first exposure occurred in older children, teenagers or adults, who did not have natural immunity. The ages affected in Calgary in the epidemics of 1952 and 1953 are shown in the graph. At these older ages, the nervous system is much more vulnerable to the virus, and paralysis is much more common. Thus, there were long-term effects of the infection which were obvious to onlookers, unlike most other infections in which full recovery was the rule.

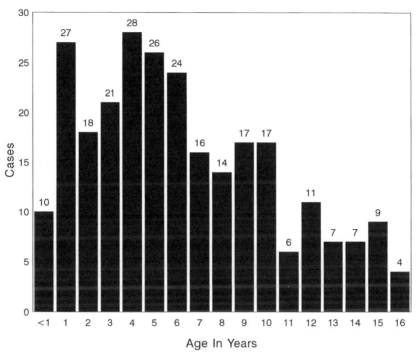

Ages of children affected with polio.
Data from Calgary Health Services.

Polio is a viral disease. Viruses are small particles, and this particular virus enters the body through the gut. It then moves along the nerves to the motor neurons of the spinal cord, the cells which control muscle movement. The official name, acute anterior poliomyelitis, reflects these facts. Poliomyelitis is derived from Greek and means "inflammation of the grey matter of the spinal cord," "polio" meaning grey and "myelo" spinal cord. One of the many names of the disease was mentioned earlier, namely infantile paralysis. Other less well-known names include paralytic poliomyelitis, non-paralytic poliomyelitis, abortive poliomyelitis. A widely known name was "the Crippler."[3]

The illness often starts with mild general malaise usually followed by an upset stomach or flu-like symptoms together with problems in moving the arms and legs, and often there is vomiting or severe diarrhea. The muscles of the neck may become stiff because of the infection of the spinal cord. These early general symptoms change, and more specific effects related to nerve damage and resultant muscle weakness appear. For example, the child might fall down with progressive paralysis, starting after the second or third day of illness. Sometimes this paralysis is only mild and hardly noticed. These changes occur as the virus invades the tissue of this child's spinal cord, destroying the nerve supplying the

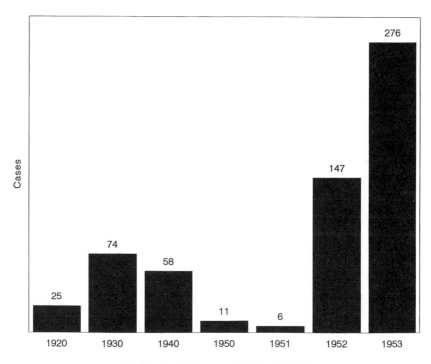

Polio in Calgary, 1921–1953.
Data from Calgary Health Services.

muscle, and messages can no longer be passed from the spinal cord to the muscles.

Later on, the effects of the disease are obvious. When there is infection of the nerves controlling the muscles in the leg, the results may be seen in the foot. For example, the toe may point downwards, because of unequal muscle use. Children with such a problem might benefit from surgical correction of the deformity or the use of braces. If the muscles surrounding the hip are affected, there will be unequal application of large muscle forces, and the hip might become dislocated. There may be spinal deformity, following the unequal effects of the disease on the large muscles in the back.

These deformities in the limbs and the back are seen in the wake of the acute illness and may remain for life. The physical consequences of polio were visible in those who survived, but many children and adults died because of complications of the disease. When paralysis affected the muscles of breathing, especially the diaphragm, the patient could not breathe. Such patients might die, and so the development of the iron lung was a major lifesaver. When the diaphragm was only slightly affected, however, the child's breathing was apparently normal. When pneumonia developed, the child was unable to cope with this additional problem, which could lead to death. In Alberta in 1937, there were 167 cases and thirteen deaths. The corresponding figures for Canada were 3,905 cases and two hundred deaths.[4] The increase in polio in Calgary from 1921 to 1953 is shown on the graph.

Although poliomyelitis reached prominence in the mid-twentieth century, it was not new. On an Egyptian tomb many thousands of years ago, a person with a withered leg thought to be due to polio is portrayed.[5]

Before the twentieth century, polio was a sporadic disease, with occasional epidemics. For example, in 1836, Sir Charles Bell reported an epidemic on the Island of Saint Helena. By the early 1900s, with a general improvement in hygiene, the characteristic seasonal epidemics occurred in the late summer and early fall, especially in North America.[6]

By 1916, the public was well aware of polio. In that year, in the U.S.A., 6,000 people died and 27,000 others were crippled. Five years later, in 1921, Franklin D. Roosevelt became the most famous patient ever to suffer from polio.[7] He was thirty-nine years old, came from a wealthy family and was politically active. He himself was vigorous and athletic, and played tennis at the family summer home. After one exhausting day of tennis and boating off the coast of New Brunswick, he developed a fever. This fever turned out to be the first sign of polio, and his legs became paralyzed. Nevertheless, he subsequently became president. He was president for four terms, a record that has not been equalled; the American Constitution has been amended to prevent anyone else being elected president for more than two terms.

Isolation was used as a means of preventing the disease. Patients diagnosed in Calgary were admitted to the Isolation Hospital for the first two weeks of illness and were strictly segregated. Parents even received information about the condition of their children indirectly by telephone and letter.[8] During the epidemics, the city issued an order prohibiting "the admission of children under the age of sixteen years to any theatre."[9]

Vaccination is another and probably more effective way of preventing infectious diseases, whether bacterial or viral. One of the first publications recording vaccination was Dr. Edward Jenner's "An inquiry into cause and effects of the *variolae vaccinae* in 1798 in England."[10] Jenner had noted that milkmaids who had had the mild illness called cowpox remained unaffected during smallpox epidemics. The Latin name for cowpox is *variolae vaccinae*, the word *vacca* meaning cow, hence the name vaccination. Jenner used this observation as a basis for his experiment. He took pus from a dairymaid who had had cowpox and vaccinated an eight-year-old boy with the material. After being exposed to smallpox, the boy did not get sick. However, this discovery was not acted on by the government. During the Franco-Prussian war of 1870, almost a century later, smallpox vaccination was again proven to be effective by an accidental experiment. The German army lost 297 men to smallpox, whereas the unvaccinated French army lost 20,000 men.[11]

In 1807, Edward Jenner heard of the smallpox problems among the Native people in Eastern Canada and sent an account of his theories and practice of vaccination to the Chiefs of the Five Nations. The chiefs were cautious at first but eventually used vaccination extensively and with enormous success. The chiefs not only thanked Jenner but sent him a string of wampum (a belt of blue native beads), the highest honor they could bestow upon their benefactor.[12]

Louis Pasteur, the famous French scientist, was interested in Jenner's ideas and worked extensively on immunization. In 1885, he produced a vaccine active against rabies. Other immunizations were developed in the nineteenth and early twentieth centuries against typhoid, diphtheria and tetanus. Routine diphtheria vaccination was introduced into Alberta in 1930, and routine tetanus vaccination in 1947.

Immunizations and Year Introduced into Alberta

Diphtheria	1930	Diphtheria, pertussis, tetanus, polio	1959
Influenza	1939	Measles – killed	1966
Pertussis	1939	Measles – live	1971
Diphtheria and pertussis combined	1943	Rubella	1971
Tetanus	1947	Smallpox – discontinued	1980
Diphtheria, pertussis and tetanus combined	1948	Measles, mumps, rubella	1982
		Hepatitis B (selected)	1983
Polio (Salk)	1956-1962	Hepatitis B (universal, grade 5)	1995
Polio (Sabin)	1962-1994	Haemophilus influenza type B (Hib)	1987
Polio with DPT and Hib	1994		

The whole issue of immunization for polio was being extensively discussed, as this was by far the best chance of control. Strictly speaking, the word "vaccination" should be applied only to smallpox, and "immunization" should be used for other diseases. However, these words are used interchangeably by most authors. It was essential that the virus be well-described and understood to allow the development of a vaccine. Progress was difficult until 1949, when J.F. Enders, F.C. Robbins and T.H. Weller of Boston were able to grow the virus in a test tube. This Nobel Prize-winning discovery enabled three major types of polio virus to be identified and studied.[13]

The effort to make a vaccine was strongly supported by the National Foundation for Infantile Paralysis, an organization set up by President Roosevelt in 1938. The March of Dimes was one of the main fundraisers for this organization. When J.E. Salk developed his vaccine, funds from the March of Dimes were used to sponsor a field trial in 1954. Connaught Laboratories (University of Toronto) produced the large amounts of vaccine required.[14] The field trial involved close to two million children, mainly in the United States of America and some in parts of Canada, including 37,406 in Alberta. These children were called "Polio Pioneers," and careful records were kept of those who received the immunization and those who developed polio. There were few who did – the vaccine was successful! The records were sent to Ann Arbor, Michigan, for analysis, those from Alberta in Box 46.[15] The Salk vaccine was an inactivated (killed-virus) vaccine. As it was up to ninety percent effective against all three types of polio virus, it was a major advance and was introduced into public use in 1955. As with most vaccines, children had to have an injection.

There are other ways of developing vaccines. One is to use a live, but weakened, virus to stimulate the body's natural process of immunity. Albert Sabin, who was born in Russia in 1906, concentrated on developing a live polio vaccine that could be swallowed. His research in the late 1950s used live virus, altered in such a way that the virus was weakened and caused a mild infection, but produced effective immunity to the powerful virus. The vaccine was first tried on a large scale in Russia in 1959, and by 1960, the vaccine was so successful that it was being used in most of the world. In 1962, Connaught Laboratories were again leaders, producing Sabin vaccine for almost four million Canadians.[16]

The dramatic success of vaccination can be seen by the contrast in the number of patients affected. Now there are no natural cases in North America; however, before 1962, 50,000 Canadians were affected and 4,000 died.[17] Canada's worst polio year was 1953, when some nine thousand cases were reported. Alberta also had its worst polio year in 1953 (139 cases and 108 deaths in the acute phase). There was a rapid fall in the number of cases, with a small epidemic in 1962, then a rapid and almost total decline.

Polio is costly to both the individual and society. Dr. Frank Mewburn[18] (an orthopaedic surgeon in Edmonton) made a number of suggestions, one of them that out-patient clinics might be more appropriate than keeping patients in hospital for a long time.[19] Despite these comments, long-term hospitalization was seen as essential although individuals had major problems affording this level of care. Private hospitals with boards had problems finding funds to treat all the patients. The Government of Alberta recognized its responsibility and implemented the *Poliomyelitis Sufferers' Act* in 1938. Under this act, all residents of Alberta suffering from the after-effects of polio had free medical, surgical and hospital care starting after two weeks of isolation in another hospital. Two Alberta hospitals were authorized to provide free treatment for polio, the University Hospital in Edmonton (which had absorbed the former Provincial Special Hospital for Infantile Paralysis built in 1927-28) and the Junior Red Cross Hospital in Calgary.[20] In 1938, because of the epidemic (167 cases in Alberta), the Minister of Health asked the Red Cross[21] for an extra twenty-six beds at the Junior Red Cross Children's Hospital (the Alberta Children's Hospital). The government gave a grant of $10.25 per day to the hospital for those admitted for treatment. Those who attended the outpatient clinics were provided splints, shoes and orthopaedic appliances free of charge. Rehabilitation assistance for those who wished to take advantage of it and even vocational training were provided. Thus there was a form of health-care service, although for one specific disease only. The acute phase of the illness was not covered by the provincial plan because it was an infectious disease; the first two weeks were the responsibility of the individual and the municipality. Other provinces had similar polio hospitalization and treatment policies, but Alberta was the first to pass legislation.

Before immunization against polio was available, during a period when there were large numbers of patients requiring treatment, enormous efforts were made to find the most effective treatment by many devoted and creative individuals. Despite these efforts, many of the treatments used in the twentieth century differ little from those described by Dr. William Osler, a famous physician in the nineteenth century. For example, in 1937, treatment seemed to be mainly rest, which was enforced by the extensive use of plaster casts in the first few weeks. It was thought necessary to restrain patients who felt so well after the onset of the disease that they started moving around too much. Subsequently, they were surprised when paralysis set in. Steel braces were commonly applied in the eighth week of the illness, after the paralysis appeared and continued until the child attained full growth.

Sister Elizabeth Kenny, an Australian nurse, made a radically different suggestion about treatment in the acute stage in 1940. She was scorned in her own country and came to the U.S.A. and also visited Canada during the 1940s. Her approach demanded a great deal of active physiotherapy, coupled by the application of hot wool packs. Indeed, these packs were so hot that many patients felt they were being scalded. Sister Kenny strongly opposed the placing of a limb in a splint, called this "alienation," and used her authority to discourage the practice.

Dr. Gordon Townsend went to Sister Kenny's clinic in Minneapolis in 1942 to study her approach. On his return, he told a story about their entrance to the Nicolet Hotel for the celebration of the contract to film Sister Kenny's life. "She was leading in her large hat and boas in all her glory, followed by a niece, several incidental retainers and finally Townsend. That was perhaps my closest approach to the seats of the mighty."[22] Following this memorable trip, Dr. Townsend brought Sister Kenny's techniques back to Calgary, for the benefit of children in the Junior Red Cross Children's Hospital.

There were many other creative treatments, and each centre had its own favorite. C.J. McSweeny visited many polio centres in 1951 and

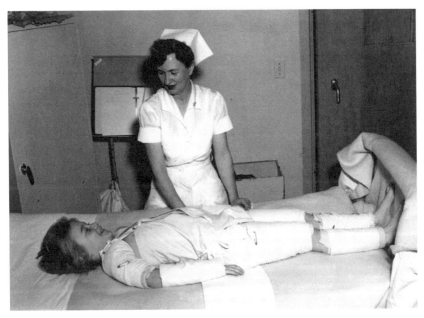

Kenny packs.

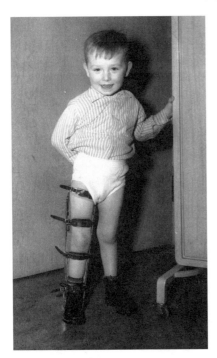

Boy with leg brace.

described many of the treatments.[23] One treatment which became popular for a short period was gamma globulin, a blood product which confers temporary immunity. Connaught Laboratories were able to fractionate the product and thus a high concentration of antibodies against polio could be obtained. Alberta received 11,000 vials of gamma globulin (at no cost) in 1953, which was given to those thought to be at high risk, to reduce spread in the large epidemic that year. Many treatments, by our standards, seem ineffective, but they were always coupled with the love and attention of the physicians and nurses and many volunteers.

Deformities of the limbs were prominent and obvious, but we should not forget the many other effects of polio such as the effect on the muscles of breathing. Some of the advances in treatment were to lead to major changes in health care. Developments stimulated by polio and its many different effects on the body were the artificial respirator, the organization we now call "critical care units" and a great emphasis on teamwork, with caregivers from many different disciplines working together to provide rehabilitation services.

The initial respirator was unlike the standard respirator in current use; called an "iron lung," it looked like a coffin! The patient was placed in the box, a tight seal was applied around the neck, then respiration was assisted by creating a negative pressure inside the box. The pressure inside the box was lower than atmospheric pressure, and therefore air was forced to enter the body through the nose and mouth. Then the negative pressure inside the body reversed, the chest relaxed, and air left the body. Iron lungs had a long history; the first was described by a Scottish physician (John Dalziel) in 1832.[24] Many others, including Alexander Graham Bell (inventor of the telephone), developed various devices. The first American tank respirator was announced in 1928, following several years work at Harvard by Philip Drinker (an engineer), Charles F. McKinnon (a paediatrician) and Louis A. Shaw (a physiologist). These iron lungs, the Drinker Machines, were well-equipped and had a number of controls.[25] The next generation, the modified Drinkers, had a sloping front and a more comfortable neck fitting. Later respirators were Emersons. John Emerson, the designer, built his first simplified respirator in 1931. It cost less than half as much as any others available at the time, operated quietly with a wide range of speeds and could be pumped manually if electricity failed. It was accepted as the standard iron lung in Canada.[26]

The regular use of these respirators eventually led to the formation of what we now call critical care units. In such units, there is specialized equipment such as ventilators and complex electronic monitoring. At least as important as the equipment is the organization of the unit with specially trained physicians and nurses present throughout the day and night who are so familiar with life-threatening illness that they can predict some crises and are available to deal with others immediately. Now critical care units are found in a wide variety of different areas. In paediatric practice, the development of neonatology and survival of many low-birth-weight infants owes much to developments in critical care. Many of the present advances that we take for granted, such as cardiac surgery, would not be possible without a dedicated critical care unit to provide post-operative care.

Patients with polio were all given high-quality care. This was the best available at the time, although knowledge about resuscitation techniques and how to provide care to a patient on a ventilator for a long time were less well developed than now. Nevertheless, teams developed that were able to work well together to help patients.

Patients with polio and their families experienced first-hand the dread

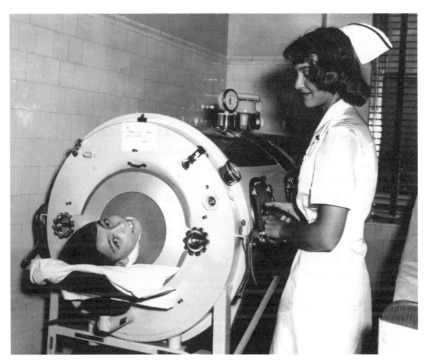

Iron lung.

society as a whole felt about this disease. They had all the anxieties of someone suffering from a disease that has an uncertain course, risk of death, and possibility of permanent deformity. The patients also had to deal with the hysteria that accompanied the epidemics and exacerbated their own anxiety. Public hysteria was increased by regular dramatic and frightening headlines in newspapers and magazines.

Despite this anxiety and exposure to hysteria and worry, patients often felt positive. They felt that their positive approach, combined with their own personal efforts, was important in leading to some degree of recovery. There was often denial of muscle weakness. Denial may have reached enormous proportions with Franklin D. Roosevelt, who, with the active collaboration of the press, presented the image of a strong, healthy man throughout his time as president of the United States of America. Indeed, a strong movement toward creating a statue of him as an invalid is only now (1997) starting.

The story of polio is not over. Although this illness can now be prevented through vaccination and natural polio is eradicated in North America, the survivors face new problems.

After many years of stability and leading an active life, during which the acute illness fades from memory, there is further progression of weakness. This development is called Post-Polio Syndrome (PPS) and appears some twenty-five to forty-five years after the original acute polio. It is estimated that between a quarter and half of all polio survivors develop PPS. The cause of this syndrome is obscure, and the sufferers have had many unpleasant experiences. They have had difficulty in finding someone who understood their problem, as most physicians today have had little experience with polio. Now research is being carried out into the late effects of polio, and there are special clinics for PPS. The effects of this syndrome on the muscles, its tendency to cause general fatigue and pain and the development of new respiratory problems are now better recognized.

Muscle weakness and fatigue are obvious. Usually the muscles affected in PPS are muscles that recovered well from the initial attack, and there may be weakness or muscle pain. The muscles affected sometimes require rest and at other times exercise. When the weakness affects abdominal muscles, there may be chronic back strain, even leading to injury. It is particularly distressing to have marked generalized fatigue after only moderate exercise or activity.

Other late effects of polio include joint or muscle pain, which has a number of causes, including osteoarthritis in the joints of the spine, inflammation around these joints and weakening of the bone (osteoporosis). Patients with polio may bear weight more on one leg than the other, which places a chronic strain on joints, and thus osteoarthritis (a wear-and-tear disease) comes on prematurely.

Respiratory muscles, which may be affected both by polio and aging, show marked deterioration. Patients with respiratory problems may have problems sleeping and develop morning headache or confusion. Their breathing may be shallow, and they may be breathless during speech. Some of these individuals require artificial help with their breathing. This may be provided in a variety of ways, one of which is the Cuirass Ventilator, a modern form of the iron lung.

From the time of its founding, the Alberta Children's Hospital played an important role in dealing with polio, especially throughout the 1940s and 1950s, and many innovative treatments were pioneered. Immunization has made the disease a rarity, but at the same time its very rarity means that parents may not understand the importance of immunization. ❖

References

1. *The State of the World's Children, 1989.* Oxford University Press, 1989.
2. *State of the World's Vaccines and Immunization.* World Health Organization, Geneva, 1996, p. 13.
3. Smith Morrow, Jane. *Patenting of the Sun: Polio and Salk Vaccines.* William Morrow and Company, Inc., New York, 1990, p. 83.
4. Rutty, C.J. *Poliomyelitis in Canada, 1927-1962.* Thesis. University of Toronto, 1995.
5. Robbins, F.C. "About the Cover Illustration," *Journal of Laboratory and Clinical Medicine*, 115(6) 1990: 770-771.

6. Paul, J.R. *Epidemiology of Poliomyelitis.* World Health Organization, Geneva, 1955, pp. 9-15.

7. Smith Morrow, Jane. *Patenting of the Sun.* p. 45.

8. Letter from the Medical Officer of Health of Calgary to a parent, July 31, 1952.

9. Letter from the Medical Officer of Health to the managers of fifteen theatres in Calgary, July 31, 1952.

10. Ackerknecht, E.H. *A Short History of Medicine.* Rev. ed., Johns Hopkins University Press, Baltimore, 1982, p. 143.

11. Jack, D. "From Circulation to Vaccination." *In Rogues, Rebels and Geniuses: The Story of Canadian Medicine.* Doubleday, Toronto, 1981, pp. 39-46.

12. Swan, R. "The History of Medicine in Canada," *Medical History,* 12 (1968): 42-51.

13. Enders, J.F., T.H. Weller and F.C. Robbins. "Cultivation of the Lansing Strain of Poliomyelitis Virus in Cultures of Various Human Embryonic Tissues." *Science* 109 (1949): 85-87.

14. Rutty, C.J. *Poliomyelitis in Canada, 1927-1962.* p. 370.

15. Smith Morrow, Jane. *Patenting of the Sun.* p. 274.

16. Rutty, C.J. *Poliomyelitis in Canada, 1927-1962.* p. 373.

17. Ibid., p. 381.

18. The Mewburn family has a long tradition of medical practice going back to 1765. Dr. Frank Mewburn's father was a founding board member of the College of Physicians and Surgeons of Alberta in 1906.

19. Mewburn, F.H. "Some Notes on After Treatment of Poliomyelitis," *Alberta Medical Bulletin,* 16:1 (February 1951): 6-8.

20. Rutty, C.J. *Poliomyelitis in Canada 1927-1962.* p. 130.

21. *Annual Report.* Calgary Branch, The Canadian Red Cross Society, 1938. [*"Annual Report"* refers to the annual reports of The Canadian Red Cross Society, Alberta Division, with a section reporting on the children's hospital.]

22. Townsend, R.G. Lecture to Orthopaedic Surgeons. October 1974. p. 13.

23. Mulder, D. "Clinical Observations on Acute Poliomyelitis," *Annals of the New York Academy of Sciences,* 753 (25 May 1995): 1-9.

24. Woollman, C.H.M. "The Development of Apparatus for Intermittent Negative Pressure Respiration (1) 1832-1918," *Anaesthesia,* 31 (1976): 537-547.

25. Markel, H. "The Genesis of the Iron Lung," *Archives of Pediatrics and Adolescent Medicine,* 148 (November 1994): 1174-1180.

26. *The Evolution of the Iron Lung.* J.H. Emerson Co., Cambridge, MA, 1978.

Further reading

Cole, W.H., and M.E. Knapp. "The Kenny Treatment of Infantile Paralysis: A Preliminary Report," *Journal of the American Medical Association,* 116 (1941): 2577-2580.

Edwards, Glen, and D. Harkness. *Life Near the Bone.* Ronalds Printing, Calgary, May 1991.

Ferguson, J.K.W. "The Story of Poliomyelitis Vaccines." *Canadian Journal of Public Health,* 55 (1964): 183-190.

Grimshaw, M.L. "Scientific Specialization and the Polio Virus Controversy in the Years Before World War II." *Bulletin of the History of Medicine,* 69(1) (Spring 1995): 44-65.

Horstmann, D.M. "The Poliomyelitis Story: A Scientific Hegira." Yale Journal of Biology and Medicine, 58(2) (March-April 1985): 79-90.

Klein, A.E. *Trial by Fury.* New York, 1992.

Kubryk, D. "Paralytic Poliomyelitis in Canada, 1960." *Canadian Medical Association Journal,* 86 (1962): 1099-1106.

Lossing, E.H. "Evaluation of Canadian Poliomyelitis Vaccination Program, 1955." *Canadian Journal of Public Health*, 47 (1956): 104-110.

Lossing, E.H. "Vaccination and the Decline in Paralytic Poliomyelitis." *Canadian Journal of Public Health*, 48 (1957): 449-453.

MacNamara, J. "Serum Therapy in Acute Poliomyelitis," *Canadian Public Health Journal*, 23 (1932): 318-326.

MacNamara, J. "The Treatment of Paralyses of Poliomyelitis." *Canadian Public Health Journal*, 23 (1932): 517-545.

McBride, E. *Crippled Children.* 2nd ed. C.V. Mosby Co. Ltd., Scarborough, Ontario, 1937.

Mulder, D. "Post Polio Syndrome – Past, Present, and Future," *The Post Polio Syndrome.* Ed. T.L. Munsat. Butterworths–Heinemann, Boston, 1991, pp. 1-8.

Nelson, A.J. "Influence of Vaccination Upon Age Distribution of Poliomyelitis." *Canadian Journal of Health*, 48 (1957): 313-316.

Paul, John R. *A History of Poliomyelitis.* Yale University Press, New Haven, 1971.

Petty, W., R.B. Winter and D. Felder. "Arteriovenous Fistula for Treatment of Discrepancy in Leg Length." *Journal of Bone Joint Surgery*, 65A (1974): 581-586.

Rice, H.V. "Poliomyelitis in Edmonton, 1953." *Alberta Medical Bulletin*, 4 (1954): 45-60.

Sabin, A.B. "Oral Poliovirus Vaccine: History of Its Development and Use and Current Challenge to Eliminate Poliomyelitis from the World." *Journal of Infectious Diseases*, 151 (1985): 420-436.

Salk, J.E. "Studies in Human Subjects on Active Immunization Against Poliomyelitis. A Preliminary Report of Experiments in Progress." *Journal of the American Medical Association*, 151 (1953): 1081-1098.

Schuler, C. "Polio Again?" *Canadian Homemakers.* Sept. 1995, pp. 86-92.

Sepples, S.B. "Polio Nursing: The Fight Against Paralysis." *Nursing Connections*, 5 (3) (Fall 1992): 31-38.

Smith, E.S.O. "A Review of the Effectiveness of Salk Vaccine in Alberta With Special Reference to the Outbreak of Poliomyelitis in 1960." *Canadian Journal of Public Health*, 52 (1961): 467-473.

Smith, E.S.O., and B.E. Cole. "A Winter Outbreak of Poliomyelitis in Northern Alberta." *Canadian Journal of Public Health*, 45 (1954): 495-501.

Varughese, P.V., A.O. Carter, S.E. Acres and J. Furesz. "Eradication of Indigenous Poliomyelitis in Canada: Impact of Immunization Strategies." *Canadian Journal of Public Health*, 80 (1989): 363-368.

Wilson, R.J., G.W.O. Moss, F.C. Potter and D.R.E. MacLeod. "Diphtheria and Tetanus Toxoids Combined with Pertussis and Poliomyelitis Vaccines," *Canadian Medical Association Journal*, 81 (1959): 450-453.

Paediatrics in Alberta: An Overview

Paediatrics is now well recognized as a medical specialty, although children are much more likely to receive medical care from family physicians than paediatricians. Throughout the history of Western medicine, physicians have been interested in the diseases of infants and children, and a few of them even spent most of their professional life dealing with this age group. However, it is only in the twentieth century that large numbers of physicians and surgeons have taken specialized training in the disorders of childhood and have made this their exclusive area of practice. Thus, the history of paediatrics in Alberta must, of necessity, deal with the history of medicine as a whole in Alberta. Further, we recognize that medicine in Alberta arose from developments within the Western medical tradition. An issue that will not be dealt with here is the role of healers in the Native tradition. Native healers in the past and today are interested in helping children and, very recently, have developed a role, albeit still small, in the Alberta Children's Hospital.

The first non-Native people who came to the Northwest Territories were fur trappers, but physicians followed soon afterwards. The early physicians were connected with the major institutions that played a role in the settlement of the West, such as the Hudson's Bay Company, the Canadian Pacific Railway and the Northwest Mounted Police (NWMP). The first Western physician in the Northwest Territories is thought to be Dr. William Todd who served in Fort Wedderburn (later known as Fort Chipewyan) as early as the 1820s.[1] He combined many duties and acted as a general administrator as well as a surgeon. Later, Dr. James Hector (from Edinburgh University in Scotland) visited Alberta (winter of 1857-58). However, he, like many others, came to explore rather than to practise medicine. He named several peaks; the name "Kicking Horse Pass" comes from an incident when he was kicked in the chest by a horse at that site. More physicians came in the latter half of the nineteenth century, such as Dr. W.M. Mackay, who arrived in 1867 and became the first president of the North Alberta Medical Society (1902) and Dr. N.J. Lindsay, who came on the first CPR passenger train and practised medicine in Calgary until 1908.[2] By 1889, there were forty medical doctors registered throughout the Northwest Territories, fourteen of them in what became Alberta. One of the few women physicians of the nineteenth century was Dr. Etta Donovan,[3] but more women came to practise in the Province of Alberta in the twentieth century.

There were only a few hospitals in Alberta in the nineteenth century, most of them little more than rooming houses. Almost all were associated with the NWMP, such as the MacLeod Hospital opened in Fort MacLeod in 1874. In Canada at that time, most physicians had an office in their own home to see patients and made home visits. There were few patients in the hospitals, which were for those with no caregivers at home. The professionals who actually provided care in the hospital were called nurses, but they had little direct training. They did have to meet general educational standards before entry, with an examination in reading, penmanship, arithmetic and English dictation.[4] In Calgary, the Calgary General Hospital opened in 1890.

The Northwest Territories Medical Association (NWTMA) was set up in 1889, when many of the physicians in the Territories had come to Banff for the annual meeting of the Canadian Medical Association. Dr. G.A. Kennedy of Fort MacLeod was elected first President of the Association, but the NWTMA did not develop into an active organization and was disbanded in 1906 when the Province of Alberta was established, at the same time the Alberta Medical Association (AMA) was formed. The first meeting of this association was held in Calgary, and the thirty-one doctors who attended elected Dr. R.G. Brett of Banff as the first President. Dr. Brett was politically active and later, as Lieutenant Governor, opened the Alberta Children's Hospital in 1922. The AMA still represents physicians within the province, as a division of the Canadian Medical Association.

Various forms of regulation of medical practitioners were introduced throughout the Western world in the second half of the nineteenth century. As part of this trend, the Government of the Northwest Territories maintained a register of physicians, and once the Province of Alberta was formed, this function was taken over by the College of Physicians and Surgeons of Alberta (CPSA), started in 1906.[5] The CPSA maintains a register, and its role is fundamentally different from that of the AMA although R.G. Brett was President of both organizations (1906-07).[6] The chief concern in the first few years was to round up irregular practitioners and unregistered doctors and address complaints of unethical conduct. In 1906, twenty-six candidates presented themselves for examination and, in the first six years, 193 were examined. After 1912, the new University of Alberta became an examining body. At the present time, all Canadian graduates take the examination for the Licence of the Medical Council of Canada (LMCC), and this is accepted by all provincial authorities. In the early days of Alberta, CPSA gave grants, two of which are of particular interest to anyone involved in paediatrics. These grants were of $5,000 in 1922 and $2,000 in 1923 to Dr. J.B. Collip to help him further his research on insulin. Also in the first two or three decades of its existence, the CPSA set fees for physicians, a function it no longer performs. The CPSA was the first provincial body in Canada to develop regulations for specialists (1926), although the only specialists recognized at that time were surgeons, and the aim of this regulation was to ensure a high standard of patient care. The CPSA remains the body responsible for licensing Alberta physicians and surgeons, but is no longer a self-governing body of physicians. It has many roles, official recognition by the government and now public representatives on the board.

The table shows the sharp increase in the number of physicians registered in Alberta more recently.[7]

ALBERTA

Year	Physicians	Specialists	
	Number	Number	Percentage
1956	1041	359	34.46
1972	2272	957	42.12
1982	3339	1504	45.04
1996	4628	2159	46.68

There were many fewer physicians registered in previous years, for example in 1941, there were still only 575 registered. There were no paediatricians when the Province of Alberta was formed. Recognition of paediatrics as a specialty came some years later from the Royal College of Physicians and Surgeons of Canada (RCPSC), founded in 1929. Originally there were only two specialties, internal medicine and surgery, but, since 1937, many specialties have been added to the list. In 1937, paediatrics, following a motion by Dr. Harold Smith Little,[8] was recognized for certification as a specialty. There were 165 paediatricians in the first group of certificants (1942-49), of which nine were from Alberta.[9] This same group of paediatricians were among the first to hold the Fellowship in Paediatrics in 1946. Now almost all paediatricians in the Province of Alberta have passed the RCPSC examination in paediatrics and hold the degree FRCPC.

However, even now in 1997, paediatricians are a small group, with approximately two hundred medical paediatricians and four paediatric general surgeons (three in Calgary) registered in the province.[10]

There were local medical societies in almost every town in Alberta, combining social functions and an opportunity for camaraderie with opportunities for continuing education and also the chance to apply political pressure on hospital managers or politicians. The Calgary Medical Society is one such local organization, which was formed in 1906 and still meets regularly. Specialized societies were formed such as the Alberta Orthopaedic Society and the Alberta Paediatric Society, which continue to exist. The Calgary Paediatric Society started as an informal offshoot of the Alberta Paediatric Society but, by 1973, wanted formal recognition to enhance its role in discussions of the Child Health Centre.[11] A formal constitution was drawn up at a time when the society was active;[12] now it has a largely social function.

The first university was established in 1906 by the Province of Alberta in the City of Strathcona (subsequently incorporated into Edmonton) and was responsible for examinations in the practice of medicine from 1912 onwards but did not provide any medical training until 1913. The first

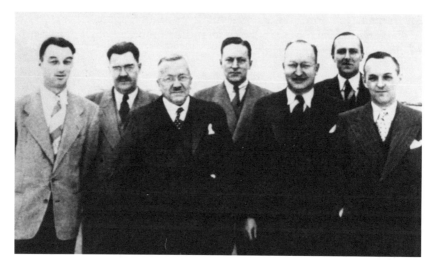

Alberta Orthopaedic Society, 1940.

medical students in Edmonton had a three-year program and then went to the University of Toronto or McGill University to complete their training. By 1921, the University of Alberta was able to offered a five-year course in medicine, and paediatrics was included as one of the subjects. The first class to complete this full course graduated in 1925, having been taught paediatrics by Dr. Douglas Leitch (1888-1974). This pioneer paediatrician graduated from the University of Toronto in 1913 and, instead of following most of his fellow graduates into general practice immediately, spent four years training in paediatrics in Toronto and New York. He served in the World War I, during which he was injured, and then came to Edmonton in 1919 to become Head of the Division of Paediatrics until 1956. He always reported to the Head of Internal Medicine at the University of Alberta, and full recognition of Paediatrics as a Department in its own right was not given by the University of Alberta until 1957.[13]

The University of Calgary Medical School is the youngest Canadian medical school and was a major stimulus for the further development of paediatrics in Calgary and Alberta. The roots of this medical school were in local and national developments. In Alberta, university education was provided solely in Edmonton until a Calgary branch of the University of Alberta was developed during World War II. There was pressure for autonomy, and, by 1964, the University of Alberta at Calgary was created, followed by The University of Calgary in 1966. By then, many wanted the new university to have a medical school using the facilities of the new hospital (Foothills). Outside Calgary, the Royal Commission on Health Services in Canada was reviewing facilities for medical education throughout Canada and thought there should be a new medical school in West-

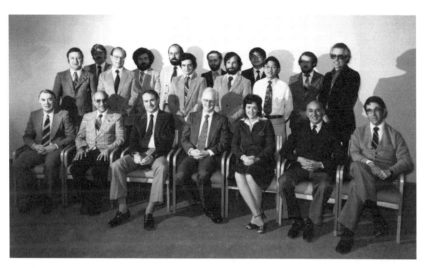

The University of Calgary Department of Paediatrics, 1981.

ern Canada, with Calgary as the best site. The University of Calgary was not enthusiastic. However, after a feasibility study confirmed that a medical school should be developed, the first Dean (Dr. W. Cochrane) was appointed (1967). Dr. Cochrane was a paediatrician (previously Head of Paediatrics at Dalhousie University) and quickly recruited a small group of faculty from many disciplines including Dr. Gerald Holman, the first Head of Paediatrics (1969). All of this early group were keen to develop new models for teaching medicine before the first group of students were admitted in 1970. The second Head of Paediatrics, Dr. R.H.A. Haslam, played an important role in leading The University of Calgary Medical School, the Alberta Children's Hospital and Foothills Hospital through the complicated negotiations that led to the transfer of acute paediatric care from the Foothills Hospital to the Alberta Children's Hospital. The Department of Paediatrics was based at Foothills Hospital in the early years, and a number of faculty members with sub-specialty interests were recruited. In 1982, the department office moved to the Alberta Children's Hospital, although neonatal paediatrics remained onsite at Foothills Hospital. When the Department of Paediatrics transferred to ACH in 1982, thirty-one of the 210 physicians were funded partly or completely by ACH at a cost of $1.4 million.[14] Dr. Haslam was succeeded by Dr. R. McArthur. He had been in Calgary for many years and concentrated on bringing together the interests of the different paediatric units within the city. The most recent Chair of Paediatrics is Dr. Grant Gall, who has an extensive research background. Dr. Gall has developed the Child Health Research Unit which concentrates on the epidemiology of childhood disease and the outcome of paediatric care. Dr. Gall has been appointed Dean of the

Faculty of Medicine in 1997, the second paediatrician to hold this post.

Research in paediatrics was identified earlier, and the planners of the 1970s thought this was important. They recognized that much research would take place at the Health Sciences Centre attached to the medical school and in association with large research groups, but supplemented this by developing the Kinsmen Research Centre at the ACH site, which focused on behavior research and genetic research and opened in 1978. Overall, research funding is acquired from many major agencies (such as the Medical Research Council and Alberta Heritage Foundation for Medical Research) and donors. Substantial funds are still supplied by the Alberta Children's Hospital Foundation and its many partners, including Children's Hospital Aid Society (CHAS) and the Kinsmen. At the present time, members of the department are awarded approximately $2 million per year for research. Research results are given prominence during the annual Child Health Research Symposium, which is open to anyone in Calgary and the surrounding area.

University training for undergraduates in Calgary was developed by a curriculum committee that ensured overall objectives for medical education were followed. The curriculum was interdisciplinary, with systems of the body taught in sequence in blocks over the first two years. Each block contains anatomy, physiology, pathology, clinical evidence of disease, diagnosis and treatment, with an emphasis on problem-oriented teaching and provision of scheduled time for independent study. There is also a continuity system to integrate information across systems. In the third and final year of the curriculum in Calgary, the "clerkship year," undergraduates attend clinical units throughout the city, which include six weeks in paediatrics with instruction on the clusters, in the Diagnostic, Assessment and Treatment Centre (DAT), and Emergency Department at the Alberta Children's Hospital, and at the Peter Lougheed Centre and Rockyview Hospitals (both for experience in the care of newborns).

All graduates in medicine require further training whether they intend to become family physicians or become a specialist in any discipline. The Alberta Children's Hospital had been involved in this post-graduate training long before The University of Calgary Medical School was established. Dr. G. Townsend approached the University of Alberta and the University of Saskatchewan to suggest that their trainees in orthopaedic surgery do a three-month rotation at the Alberta Children's Hospital, under the supervision of Dr. Glen Edwards (Director of Post-graduate Studies). The first residents from Saskatchewan came in 1961, and by the next year, the rotation had been increased to six months. By the end of the 1960s, the affiliation with the University of Saskatchewan faded. During the time this rotation was in existence, the teaching was innovative, including a seminar one evening per week for three hours at the start of the program and an expectation that residents attend Orthopaedic Rounds which had been started in 1948 by Dr. G. Townsend, Dr. M. Cody and Dr. Cyril Walsh-Smyth.

The Residency Training Program in Paediatrics was approved by the Royal College of Physicians and Surgeons of Canada in 1970. The early records do not clearly separate those in paediatrics from other programs, but there were sixteen interns in 1969-70 and twenty-six in 1970-71. Of the twenty-one interns in 1972-73, one was assigned to paediatrics. For twelve years, most of this training was in the acute paediatric units at the Foothills Hospital. On one review of the program by the Royal College of Physicians and Surgeons, there was severe criticism of the split between Foothills Hospital and the Alberta Children's Hospital and a suggestion that the Alberta Children's Hospital be on the Health Sciences site.[15] Later in the 1970s, some residents occasionally came to the Alberta Children's Hospital to participate in the care of children with chronic disorders attending the DAT Centre. In the first full year at ACH (1982-83), there were twenty-four residents, six of whom later joined the ACH staff.

Dr. Joel Fagan was the first Director of the training program, then Dr. Diane Morrison was recruited to the Department of Paediatrics in 1979 and was Program Director from 1981 to 1991. She was succeeded by Dr. Taj Jadavji who has overseen many developments in paediatric education. External reviews of the program have been complimentary, and the number of candidates from all over Canada who apply to join the program attest to its high quality. Residents from Saudi Arabia and other overseas countries, who will eventually return to their own country, are trained in Calgary. Several hold leadership positions in paediatrics in Saudi Arabia. There are also sub-specialty programs within Paediatrics including Nephrology, Gastroenterology, Respirology, Infectious Disease and Neonatology. The Royal College of Physicians and Surgeons of Canada originally thought that adult and paediatric sub-specialties would have the same training and examination,[16] but now there is full support for the concept that paediatric sub-specialty training follows general paediatric training and merits its own certification process.

Paediatric surgeons are an important part of paediatric care but, academically, are members of the Department of Surgery. However, all of the paediatric surgeons work closely with paediatricians and give considerable service to education and research at the Alberta Children's Hospital. Post-graduate education in surgery continues for trainees in orthopaedic surgery, general surgery, plastic surgery and neurosurgery. In general, trainees in these areas rotate through the Alberta Children's Hospital for part of their training. There is also a training fellowship in orthopaedic surgery so anyone interested in the paediatric aspects can complete their training within Calgary.

The community paediatricians of the 1960s and early 1970s made major contributions to the development and early growth of The University of Calgary Department of Paediatrics. In their early years, many of them combined private practice in paediatrics with some sub-specialty care and also pressed for the recruitment of fully trained specialists and further development of subspecialty areas. Later specialists came in a joint academic and clinical role, with funding from university and hospital budgets. There has always been mutual recognition that academic physicians and community physicians alike have an important role in paediatric care, and so tension between "town and gown" factions has been minimal in Calgary. Many community paediatricians continue to give valuable service in the DAT Centre and other specialty areas. For example, Dr. R. Truscott was a general paediatrician in private practice with additional training in oncology and has worked in that department from the time of his arrival in Calgary. He continued to be involved in this department and has actively participated in the development of oncology.

Continuing medical education is a major activity at the Alberta Children's Hospital, as it is recognized that education does not stop once a specialty qualification has been achieved. This is provided in co-operation with The University of Calgary and other bodies for family physicians, paediatricians and many other health-care professionals. There are seminars, workshops and lectures, all with the aim of ensuring that professionals remain up to date in knowledge and practice.❖

References

1. Jamieson, H.C. "Early Medicine in Alberta, the First Seventy-Five Years." Canadian Medical Association, Alberta Division, 1947, p. 2.
2. Humbes, D.M. *What's in a Name? Calgary*. City of Calgary, 1995, p. 99.
3. Jamieson, H.C. "Early Medicine in Alberta, the First Seventy-Five Years." p. 138.
4. Ibid., p. 89.
5. Ibid., p. 53.
6. First Registrar-Treasurer of the College of Physicians and Surgeons of Alberta was Dr. J.D. Lafferty and the Council was Dr. E.A. Braithwaite (Edmonton), Dr. J.M. Hodson (Strathcona), Dr. W. Simpson (Lacombe), Dr. R.G. Brett (Banff), Dr. G.A. Kennedy (MacLeod) and Dr. F.H. Mewburn (Lethbridge).
7. Data supplied by the College of Physicians and Surgeons of Alberta.
8. *Minutes*. Council of the Royal College of Physicians and Surgeons of Canada, October 29, 1937.
9. First certificants in Paediatrics in Alberta (1942-49): Edmund Cairns (Lethbridge), James Calder (Edmonton), Pearl Christie-Dowling (Calgary), Morley Cody (Calgary), Douglas Leitch (Edmonton), Harold Price (Calgary), George Prieur (Calgary), Helen Reid (Edmonton), Gordon Swallow (Edmonton).
10. Data supplied by the College of Physicians and Surgeons of Alberta.
11. Correspondence from Dr. M.C. Caldwell to the Alberta Medical Association, February 22, 1973.
12. *Minutes*. Calgary Paediatric Society, February 7, 1973.
13. Chairs, Department of Paediatrics, University of Alberta: Dr. J. Kenneth Martin, 1957-68, Dr. Ernest E. McCoy, 1971-84, Dr. Peter Olley, 1986-96.
14. Bonham, A. *Review of Medical Services*, Alberta Children's Hospital, 1983.
15. *Minutes*. Division of Paediatrics, University of Calgary, September 9, 1975.
16. Graham, J.H. Letter from RCPSC Secretary to Dr. J.K. Martin, August 7, 1970.

Further reading

Chumak, S.Z., ed. *The Spirit of Alberta*. The Alberta Heritage Foundation, Edmonton, 1978.

Edwards, Glen, and D. Harkness. *Life Near the Bone*. Ronald's Printing, Calgary, 1991.

Hamowy, R. *Canadian Medicine: A Study in Restricted Entry*. Fraser Institute, Toronto, 1984.

Lower, J.A. Arthur, and D.Z. McIntyre. *Western Canada*. Vancouver, 1983.

McDougall, Gerald M., ed. *Teachers of Medicine: The Development of Graduate Medical Education in Calgary*. University of Calgary, 1987.

McKendry, J.B.J., and J.D. Bailey. *Paediatrics in Canada*. Canadian Paediatric Society, Ottawa, 1990.

McPhedran, N. Tate. *Canadian Medical Schools*. Harvest House, Montreal, 1993.

Palmer, H. *Alberta, a New History*. Hurtig, Edmonton, 1990.

Still, G.S. *The History of Paediatrics*. Oxford University Press, 1931.

Taylor, W.C., and H.B. Armstrong. *History of the Department of Paediatrics, University of Alberta, 1919 to 1992*. Department of Paediatrics, Edmonton, 1993.

Nursing in Alberta Through the Years

During part of the nineteenth century and most of the twentieth century, nursing was thought to exemplify feminine characteristics of altruism and service. This is supported by a look at the origin of the word "nursing" which is based on "to nourish" and denoted a wet nurse, a woman who "nourished" or breastfed someone else's child. By 1590, the word "nurse" came to mean a woman who looked after the sick.[1] Today, the verb "to nurse" denotes breastfeeding as well caring for the sick. Because of these characteristics, nursing and teaching, have been considered appropriate occupations for women who wished to work outside the home. Today, nurses are held in high regard in society, and it is recognized that the profession demands a high level of educational preparation, with an ever-increasing skill level.

In the early part of the last century, women who were nurses were usually women off the street, constantly drunk, very dirty and with little knowledge, particularly not medical. The only training for nurses was through a religious order. Florence Nightingale was the person who changed that situation. She envisioned nursing as a highly disciplined occupation with its own code of conduct; nurses received a well-rounded education to care for patients properly. She was also an epidemiologist and a researcher, and the meticulous notes she kept on her patients demonstrated the huge difference her methods made in dramatically lowering the morbidity rate of soldiers in the Crimean War. Her book *Notes on Nursing* was published in 1859 and dealt almost exclusively with home nursing. Shortly after the book was published, she started the first school of nursing for lay women in association with St. Thomas Hospital in London.[2] Only women could register in this school, and its existence was not dependent on the financial well-being of the hospital. Some of these concepts became lost as new hospital schools were founded all around the world,[3] but at least nursing was elevated to a level which reflected a suitable and respectable occupation for women.

The first visiting nurses in Canada belonged to a religious order called the Sisters of Charity of Montreal, formed in 1738 by Marguerite d'Youville based on the model of St. Vincent de Paul.[4] The color of the habit gave rise to the popular name, Grey Nuns. These were all women of suitable character and background recruited from France and then trained in Quebec. From the beginning, these nurses cared for anyone regardless of race or creed, both nursing and educating people on hygiene. They entered patients' homes unlike other orders of nuns who were not permitted to venture into the community. The Grey Nuns were also the first nurses and actually the first non-Native women[5] to arrive in Alberta. They came to

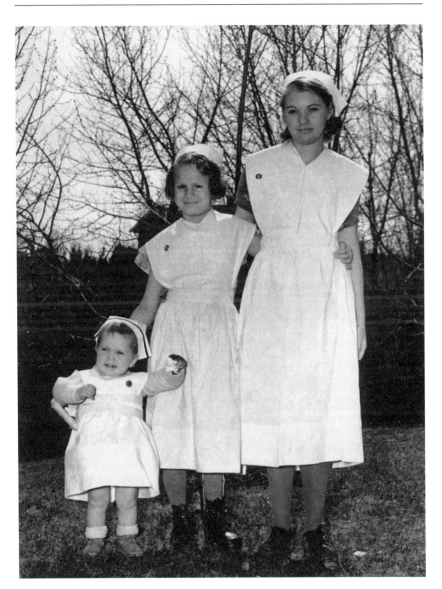

"I want to be a nurse."

support Father Lacombe in 1859 and established the first hospital in 1881 in the St. Albert mission near Edmonton.[6] Thus a system of rudimentary health care was already in place before most of the settlers arrived. In Calgary, the Grey Nuns established the Holy Cross Hospital in 1891.

At the same time as the religious orders were providing nursing care in Alberta and elsewhere in North America, some of the Nightingale ideas crossed the Atlantic. The first North American school of nursing[7] was not established until 1873 in Bellevue Hospital in New York. One year later, the first Canadian school was started in association with St. Catharine's General Hospital in Ontario. The admission standards were "plain English education, good character and Christian motives." The first training school for nurses in Alberta was founded in 1894 in Medicine Hat General Hospital (itself opened in 1890). Training in all of these institutions was by apprenticeship in the hospital, and lectures were privileges, attended only when hospital duties allowed. As the trainee nurses were hired for little money, they more or less subsidized the hospital, and their main role was to sustain the operations of the hospital itself. The Medicine Hat Nursing School was open to all interested ladies, whether or not they wished to become nurses, and this certainly illustrates the fact that nursing was seen as a regular part of a woman's life in caring for the health of others. The training at that hospital school emphasized the development of personal qualities such as altruism and dedication, instead of the traditional educational objectives such as acquisition of knowledge or ability to think and reason. These early nurses often provided the only medical service in Alberta. In the early days, the only physicians were in towns such as Fort MacLeod and Calgary, and as more physicians arrived, they generally took a leadership role. This was in keeping with the perception that nursing did not involve independent thinking or decision making. Nursing was an art, and the notion that it was a science came much later. Indeed, it is only in the last few decades that this aspect has become more firmly established through scholarships and research.

The Victorian Order of Nurses (VON), a national, volunteer and philanthropic organization founded in 1897 also provided home nursing and public health nurses. The national founder was Lady Ishbel Aberdeen, wife of the governor-general (1893-98), and the founders of the Alberta Chapter (1909) were Henrietta Muir Edwards, James Lougheed and Isabella Lougheed. The VON nurses had a full basic training, additional training in midwifery, and six months training in district nursing in training schools established all over Canada. Their scope was home visiting and educating the public on the principles of hygiene, food preparation, and so on, and sometimes, when home visits were not possible, cottage hospitals were established. In the prairie provinces, the VON came to mean both hospital nursing and home visiting nursing. The hospitals they founded were turned over to the community as soon as possible, the last one being in 1924. Once publicly funded health units were established, the VON concentrated on home visiting, a service they still provide. They developed community-based nursing in Canada and were among the first to offer scholarships to their nurses to take the degree in public health nursing as soon as it was available.[8]

Public health nursing had a different role from home nursing and also has a long history. The importance of public health is recognized by the current location of the Scarborough Health Unit physically within the premises of the Alberta Children's Hospital, although this close connection with the hospital has not always been the case. Baby Wellness Clinics were started in Calgary in 1922, but they had no connection with the Alberta Children's Hospital. Prevention was not a major function of the hospital. Moreover, the hospital itself had the role of looking after orthopaedic in-patients and out-patients. Sick children were looked after in the other hospitals. However, many recognized the importance of public health nurses and their focus on prevention, long before 1922. Prevention was recognized by legislation in Ontario in 1884, which established a public health organization and sanitary codes. The Board of Health could, for example, issue quarantine orders as one way to fight an infectious disease. After World War I, the Canadian Red Cross Society established as one of its goals the facilitation of public health through the training of nurses, and this training became the driving force for the establishment of nursing courses at some Canadian universities. Women's organizations, as they demanded better health care for their members and their children, supported the establishment of a program of sending trained nurses into isolated areas. There were travelling clinics for examinations and treatment, and payment was often in the form of goods. This service was modified as communities developed their own health services and started hiring physicians and nurses. When Alberta became a province in 1905, it also recognized the importance of public health service. At first it was part of the Department of Agriculture,[9] but later a Public Health Nursing Service was established (1917), a public health branch in 1918, and a department within the government (the Department of Public Health) in 1919.[10]

Throughout the twentieth century, there has been increasing recognition that many issues can only be looked at on a collective level by the governments of provinces and countries. Thus, public health remains an important branch of government and has as its main role the promotion of health and the prevention of illnesses.

Nursing care of the sick was developing in Alberta at the same time as public health nursing. Nursing care, however, was given at home, although this depended on being able to afford it, as a hospital was only for the less well off. Later, as scientific medicine developed, hospitals changed from a charity institution or Alms House into a centre of nursing and medicine. For a large part of this century, many nurses seemed willing to sacrifice personal life for their work, as they encountered poor working conditions and extremely long hours. In the 1910s, student nurses were expected to work twelve hours a day with only half a day off per week. Their tasks were all-encompassing, including dusting and cleaning, and such job descriptions are in the *Nursing Procedures Book* of the late 1930s of the Alberta Children's Hospital. All hospitals found it cheaper to have trainee nurses do these jobs rather than hire people for the task. The hospitals were staffed largely by students, who, after graduating, had great difficulty finding jobs caring for patients in their home. Many of the nurses at that time were keen to have graduate nurses established as primary providers of nursing care in hospital.

In the early part of the century, the responsibilities of the jobs of these trainee nurses would depend on the particular setting. For example, in a hospital where physicians were present much of the time, tasks might be "domestic," although domestic and therapeutic functions are often embedded in the simplest of tasks. In hospitals such as the Alberta Children's Hospital which provided convalescent care, there was probably much more independence for the nurses, as the physicians only checked patients infrequently. As the science and technology of nursing has developed, more skills are required from nurses, and they have often taken over procedures from physicians, once these have become well established. Many nurses in practice today remember that the administration of intravenous medication was at one time done only by physicians, and even today in many parts of the world, these functions are still performed only by physicians.

There was a sudden increase in the demand for the services of nurses with a wave of new hospitals. This trend started after World War II (1939–45) and was further stimulated by the *Hospital Insurance and Diagnostic Services Act* of 1957, which was implemented in Alberta in 1958, when the province became responsible for the building and maintenance of hospitals. The final steps in developing the national system of health insurance was the *Medical Care Act* of 1968. Later, in the 1960s, many specialized areas in the hospital developed, and there was an acute shortage of nurses. In the 1950s and 1960s, married nurses were actively hired to go back into the work force.

The development of more jobs for nurses made the need for an organization to represent them more urgent, although there had been formal organizations of nurses from the late nineteenth century. In Canada, the Canadian Society of Superintendents of Training Schools for Nurses was formed in 1907, and in 1908 the Provisional Society of the Canadian National Association of Trained Nurses was formed in Canada, later to become the Canadian Nurses Association (CNA). The Canadian Nurses' Foundation is linked to the CNA and provides scholarships, bursaries and fellowships for graduate training. From 1962 to 1987, 244 Master Awards and sixty-six Doctoral Awards were granted.[11]

The Calgary Association of Graduate Nurses was formed in 1904; one of its main goals was to pass provincial legislation for the registration of nurses. They were successful in 1916 with the passage of the *Registered Nurses' Act* which legally acknowledged a level of care and gave status and credibility to nurses in Alberta. The Alberta Association of Graduate

Nurses was formed and, in 1920, became the Alberta Association of Registered Nurses (AARN). The first forty years were characterized by intensive activity to make the profession viable and respected.[12] The large number of nurses and the new government-controlled hospitals needed ways to bargain for wages and conditions. At first, the AARN bargained on behalf of its members, but eventually the conflicts in a dual role were recognized and the AARN withdrew from bargaining in 1977.[13] The United Nurses of Alberta became the main bargaining organization in the province. There was a strike in 1979 which had an impact on ACH, although nurses there were not on strike. The *Health Services Act* in 1982 made it illegal for nurses to go on strike, as they were deemed to perform an essential service. There was, however, a province-wide nineteen-day strike in 1988, immediately before the Olympics,[14] as the nurses sought, among other issues, an increase in pay of ten percent. This strike, while distressing to all involved, may have helped some of the nurses at ACH to come together. This was one of the few activities that nurses from the DAT Centre and in-patient nurses participated in together. During that strike, some services continued, with the agreement of the UNA. The nurses criticized many government decisions, such as the construction of the Peter Lougheed Centre at a cost of $110 million. The United Nurses of Alberta remains a strong force in negotiation for the nurses with the employers, and indeed there was almost a strike in 1997. The AARN remains the main body responsible for registration and maintenance of standards of nursing.

The training of nurses has changed extensively, but even at the time of introduction of medicare, there was still an apprenticeship approach. Slowly the realization came that nurses' training should be part of the general educational system. In the Alberta Children's Hospital, nurses had a broad general training, which included orthopaedic nursing. Orthopaedic nurses got their main training on the job, reinforced by lectures from physicians. Margaret Baxter changed much of this at ACH. She herself had university training in orthopaedic nursing in Boston before she became Director of Nursing in 1951. She realized that ACH offered unique conditions for the initiation of a formal student nurse program. For example, patients from all over the southern part of Alberta, and sometimes from out of province, came to the hospital, and thus there was a wealth of educational opportunities. She implemented a program where student nurses from Lethbridge Municipal Hospital, Medicine Hat General Hospital, Holy Cross Hospital and Calgary General Hospital came for a six-week period of orthopaedic training. These nurses stayed at the hospital under the supervision of a house-mother, Edna Stout, and all the student nurses wore the uniform of their school, all with different colors and different caps. Phyllis Weir was responsible for educational aspects and supervision on the nursing unit. Before taking

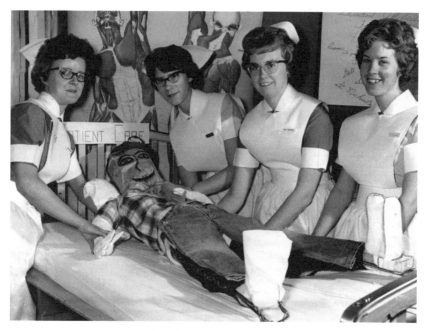

Students practising.

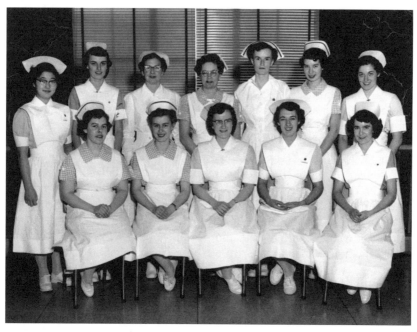

Each school had a distinct cap.

up her position, she also went on a course in orthopaedic nursing at Boston University. Once she returned, she used dolls to explain the different sorts of tractions and frames used in orthopaedic nursing. Regular lectures were part of the course for student nurses and also for staff nurses, who were given opportunities for further growth.

Later, in the 1950s and 1960s, as the work week was reduced to forty-nine hours, it was acknowledged that a trainee nurse should have dedicated time for education, and thus the block system was started. In this system of training, there is a block of formal training, alternating with a block of practical training. At the same time, there was discussion on the optimal site of nursing education. Should this be in the hospitals' schools, with the danger that the needs of the hospital might come before the needs of education, or in a college or university setting? All hospital schools had been closed by the end of the 1960s in some Canadian provinces, and in Calgary, Mount Royal College established the first diploma nursing program outside a hospital in 1967. This program continues. The University of Alberta first established a Masters of Nursing Program in 1975 and required a strong research component. The first students in the Bachelor of Nursing Program at The University of Calgary were accepted in 1970, and the first Master's Program was started in 1981.

The Alberta Task Force on Nursing Education stimulated many developments and, in 1975, stated that by 1995 all entrants to practice should have a university degree, although this was later amended to the year 2000. Although these recommendations were only for new nurses starting training, they had a major influence on existing registered nurses, many of whom have returned to university to complete their education. The Alberta Children's Hospital offers competitive scholarships to allow those with the qualification RN to go to university for a Bachelor of Nursing degree. Beyond this, it is now recognized that today's graduate is a beginning practitioner, and that lifelong learning is the rule. The impact of technology and changing roles requires constant development of knowledge and different skills.

The funding and administrative responsibility for hospital schools was transferred in 1983 from the departments of Hospitals and Medical Care and Social Services and Community Health to the Department of Advanced Education. It has not been easy to develop agreement on a curriculum for nursing, but the University of Alberta Faculty of Nursing and Red Deer College were the first to plan an innovative collaborative program for an integrated degree. They started in 1990. Calgary followed with a conjoint program between the Faculty of Nursing, Foothills Hospital and Mount Royal College in 1993 with the paediatric component at the Alberta Children's Hospital, with part-time clinical instructors.

The University of Alberta has also pioneered the distance delivery of its post-RN degree programs through the use of modern telecommunica-

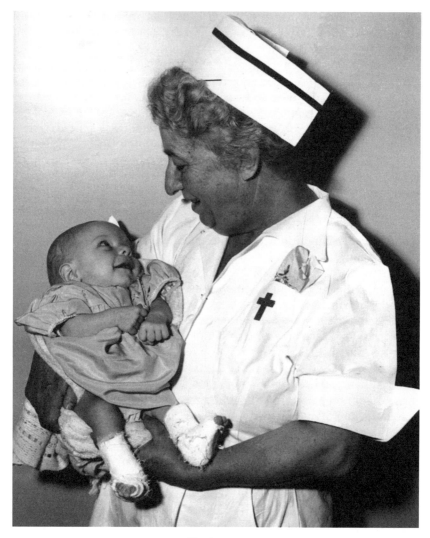

Caring....

tions since 1985. Thus nurses may practice their profession and work toward a degree simultaneously in programs at the universities of Alberta, Calgary, Lethbridge and Athabasca. The University of Alberta Faculty of Nursing, in concert with The University of Calgary Faculty of Nursing, established a doctoral program in 1991, the first in Canada, and now nurses do not need to go to the United States for this further degree. The approach to program planning is midway between the U.S.A. (extensive course work) and Great Britain (self-study, little course work).[15] The doctoral program is important for the development of the nursing profession, and it allows research programs to be combined with an academic appointment in nursing. It prepares nurses to contribute to the expanding knowledge of theory and research behind nursing and thus ultimately to improvement of care for patients. There is no structured post-doctoral study. The one exception is the Alberta Foundation for Nursing Research which established a post-doctorate (funding) category. [16]

The rate of entry of men into the predominantly female profession has been quite slow compared to the rate of entry of women into professions traditionally for men. Some of the obvious barriers were the perception that caring was a female job, and men were often excluded from nursing schools. When they were included, they were not allowed to do the entire training. For example, until the 1970s male nursing students were not permitted to study the practice and theory of obstetrics and gynaecology.[17] It will be interesting to see if there is an increasing number of men joining the profession of nursing in the next few years, as the profession undergoes further changes.

The rapid expansion of the profession of nursing, along with the rapid expansion of hospitals, came to a halt in the 1990s. Within the cutbacks and changes, there has been a strong focus to shift health care from care in the hospital to care at home. Now many will see a return of nursing care to its roots. Nurses, however, will continue to be important partners in the professional health-care team, whether in the hospital or at home. Overall, nurses are likely to take on greater roles; for example, new positions such as nurse practitioners are being developed. Many of these developments occur at the Alberta Children's Hospital where there is strong support for the continuing professional development of nurses and a strong desire on the part of the nurses to be as well prepared as possible.❖

References

1. Little, W., et al. *The Shorter Oxford Dictionary*. 3rd ed., Vol. 2, Oxford, Clarendon Press, 1972.
2. Kerr, J.R., and J. MacPhail. *Canadian Nursing Issues and Perspectives*. 2nd ed., C.V. Mosby Co. Ltd., Scarborough, Ontario, 1991, p. 69.
3. Ibid., p. 232.
4. Ibid., pp. 8-9.
5. Cashman, Tony. *Heritage of Service: The History of Nursing in Alberta*. Alberta Association of Registered Nurses, Commercial Printers Ltd., Edmonton, 1966, p. 5.
6. Kerr, J.R., and J. MacPhail. *Canadian Nursing Issues and Perspectives*, p. 16.
7. Ibid., p. 233.
8. Baumgart, A., and J. Larsen, eds. *Canadian Nursing Faces the Future*, 2nd ed., Times Mirror Professional Publishing, Markham, Ontario, 1992, pp. 611-626.

9. McHutchion, Diane. *Early Community Health Nursing in Alberta.* Alberta Association of Registered Nurses . 49(10) (1993): 11-12.
10. The department of the Government of Alberta responsible for hospitals and health has had many different names, and responsibilities have changed over the years.

Department of Public Health	1919–1967
Department of Health	1968–1971
Alberta Health & Social Development	1971–1974
Alberta Social Services & Community Health	1974–1986*
Alberta Community & Occupational Health	1986–1988*
Alberta Hospitals and Medical Care	1978–1988*
Alberta Health	1988 to date

*Some overlap

11. Kerr, J.R., and J. MacPhail. *Canadian Nursing Issues and Perspectives*, p. 340.
12. Ibid., p. 263.
13. Baumgart, A., and J. Larsen, *Canadian Nursing Faces the Future*, 1992, p. 566.
14. Ibid., p. 586.
15. Kerr, J.R., and J. MacPhail. *Canadian Nursing Issues and Perspectives*, pp. 436-437.
16. Ibid., p. 438.
17. Ibid., p. 71.

Further reading

Hardwick, E., E. Jameson and E. Tregillus. *The Science, the Art and the Spirit: Hospitals, Medicine and Nursing in Calgary*. Century, Calgary, 1975.

Kerr, J.C. Ross. Prepared to Care: Nurses and Nursing in Alberta. Thesis, University of Alberta, Edmonton, 1996.

Kwasny, Barbara, ed. *Nuns and Nightingales*. Alumni Association of Holy Cross School of Nursing, Calgary, 1982.

Masson, Madeleine. *A Pictorial History of Nursing*. Hamlyn, Twickenham, 1985.

Peach, J. *Days Gone By*. Fifth House, Saskatoon, 1993.

Peach, J. *Thanks for the Memories*. Fifth House, Saskatoon, 1994.

Schartner, A. *Health Units of Alberta*. Health Unit Association of Alberta. Co-op Press, Edmonton, 1982.

Stewart, Irene. *These Were Our Yesterdays: A History of District Nursing in Alberta*. Friesen Printers, Calgary, 1979.

PART TWO

THE FIRST HOSPITAL 1922-1929

❖❖❖❖❖❖❖❖❖❖❖❖❖❖

The Red Cross and Brickburn House

There is a large red cross in mosaic stones in the floor outside the library on the second floor of the Alberta Children's Hospital in front of the elevators. Those walking over the cross may have many different destinations. Nowadays, one direction leads to the Ophthalmology Department, another to Mental Health and Family Resources. A corridor also leads to the 1982 extension of the Alberta Children's Hospital. In the floor, there is tangible recognition of the role of the Red

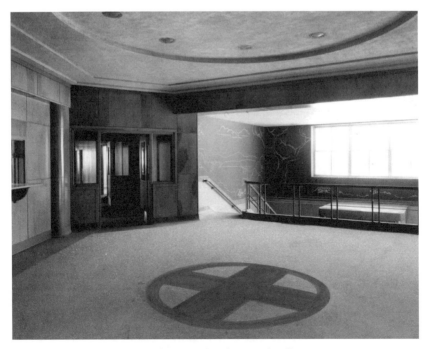

The red cross in the main floor.

Cross in developing what was to become the Alberta Children's Hospital. The actual cross was present in the previous building and is a physical link with the past.

The beginnings of the Red Cross were on a different continent in the mid-nineteenth century. Henry Dunant from Switzerland was instrumental in the foundation of the Red Cross. He had also heard of the newly founded British Association called the Young Men's Christian Association (YMCA), and when he was only twenty-one years old, he founded the Young Men's Christian Union in Geneva as the Swiss counterpart of the British organization.[1] He wanted this to be a global non-sectarian movement, and it became the worldwide organization still known as the YMCA.[2] When he was thirty years old, he witnessed the devastating battle of Solferino (Italy) on June 24, 1859, between Austria and France.[3] He crossed the battlefield and saw that there were dying and wounded everywhere. There were said to be nearly 40,000 wounded men,[4] the total dead and wounded being approximately 80,000 to 100,000.[5] Dunant organized aid for the wounded and did as much as he could do personally to relieve the suffering. He did not distinguish between friends or enemies as he offered help. This concept, taken up by the Women of Castiglione, was expressed *Tutti fratelli* (all are brothers).[6]

Henry Dunant published a book in 1862 in which he not only described these experiences, but also made a strong appeal to establish foreign relief societies. These societies, developed and trained in times of peace, would be ready to give care to the wounded in wartime, regardless of nationalities.[7] His vision was "an appeal to be made to men of all countries and of all classes..., for all can, in one way or another, each in his own sphere and within his own limitations, do something to help the good work forward. Such an appeal is to be made to ladies as well as men...."[8] Henry Dunant also suggested, "an international principle, sanctioned by a Convention which would serve as the basis of the support for the relief societies." This vision inspired internationally well-connected humanitarian men, and in 1863, thirty-six dignitaries representing sixteen countries met in Geneva. They recommended the formation of national committees for the relief of military wounded. During the Geneva Convention in 1864, an international treaty that set rules for the alleviation of suffering of soldiers was signed by twelve governments.[9]

The First International Conference of the Red Cross was held in 1867, attended by nine governments and sixteen national committees.

The Swiss played such a major role in developing this new code of wartime conduct that their flag was honored.[10] The colors of the Swiss national flag were reversed to become a red cross on a white field, and this is still the symbol of the Red Cross Society.[11]

The vision of Henry Dunant has been fulfilled many times over, and, in 1997, it is evident how successful his vision has been and what a

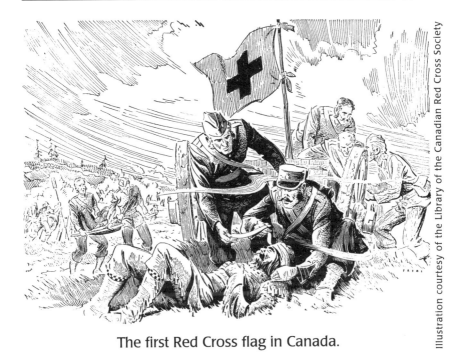

Illustration courtesy of the Library of the Canadian Red Cross Society

The first Red Cross flag in Canada.

tremendous impact it has had all over the world. There are more than 165 national Red Cross Societies and between 250 and 300 million members worldwide.[12] The Red Cross Youth Section (individuals from ten to eighteen years of age) itself has 50 million members.[13]

The first Nobel Prize for Peace was awarded jointly to Henry Dunant and the French activist Frederic Passy. The citation for Dunant's prize read: "It must ever be borne in mind that Dunant's vision was not that of a single nation, but he looked upon the world as a whole. He was one of the great apostles of the doctrine of the brotherhood of man." This visionary made enemies and he had no role in the organization after 1867.[14]

The Red Cross is now so familiar that it is almost as if the symbol has been used forever. The first use of this emblem in Canada was in 1885 by Dr. G. Sterling Ryerson, the Surgeon-General, during the Riel rebellion. He called it "a Geneva Red Cross on a flag of factory cotton,"[15] explaining that it was made from an old flour sack, the cross in turkey red being roughly stitched on.[16] This red material was said to have come from a recruit's red flannel underwear.[17] Dr. Ryerson's dedication and energy led to the formation of the Canadian Branch of the British Red Cross Society in 1896.[18]

The Canadian Red Cross was active overseas throughout World War I. The European activities were co-ordinated from headquarters in London, England. A Red Cross hospital was set up near London for Canadian soldiers injured in Europe. This hospital was built near Taplow on the

Cliveden Estate, which belonged to the Astor family. In 1914, Dr. F.H.H. Mewburn was in charge of the surgical suite there. At the end of the first world war, this hospital was pulled down, and the land returned to the family.

A new hospital opened on the same estate on June 5, 1940. This hospital cost $1 million, and at the time of opening had six hundred beds. The opening ceremony attracted many guests, including R.B. Bennett, the former Canadian prime minister who had retired to Britain and represented the Canadian Red Cross.[19] The staff was Canadian, and all of the supplies in that Second-World-War hospital were also Canadian, including bed clothes, bandages and so on. Maple furniture and the mattresses were made in Canada and brought to England. The hospital included a research laboratory led by Sir Frederick Banting, the co-discoverer of insulin. He was an enthusiastic expert on the new specialty of aviation medicine. In 1941, he was insistent he get to Britain as soon as possible with new medical knowledge, and he wanted to be there for the invasion of Europe which was thought to be eminent. His plane crashed off the east coast of Newfoundland, February 24, 1941, and he was killed.[20]

After World War II, the Canadian Red Cross Society donated this hospital to the British people. It was designed as a research hospital and was called the Canadian Red Cross Memorial Hospital. It concentrated on juvenile rheumatism and became a worldwide centre under the leadership of Professor E.G.L. Bywater initially, and later Dr. Barbara Ansell. The Canadian Red Cross Memorial Hospital was closed in 1983, despite a large public campaign to keep it open.

World War I was responsible for many changes throughout the Western world. At the end of the war, the Covenant of the League of Nations, part of the Treaty of Versailles, crystallized the goals of the Red Cross, namely, "the improvement of health, the prevention of disease and the mitigation of suffering throughout the world."[21] This was signed by Canada, as an independent country, although the Canadian Red Cross did not become independent from the British Red Cross until 1927.[22] Many different societies were combined in the league of Red Cross Societies, including Islamic societies whose emblem was a red crescent on a white field. A peace program was formulated which would become relevant to events in Calgary.

The peace program was idealistic and had a number of different goals. The major goals were to hold a public health campaign and to work for disabled veterans and their families. There was a dedication to restoring health and vigor for young, crippled Canadians. The Red Cross wished to establish outpost hospitals and to welcome new Canadians. They also wanted to start home nursing in rural districts and to be ready in any calamity or disaster. The new mandate to prevent illness led to the Faculty of Nursing and Health at the University of British Columbia in 1919.[23]

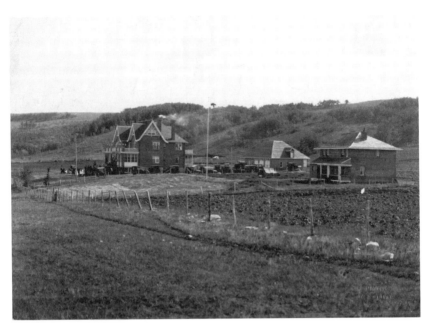

Brickburn House, Sarcee Road S.W.

The Canadian Red Cross operated on a national and international level during World War I. Its purpose was to recruit, train and supervise volunteers working to help Canadian servicemen in hospitals, in the field of battle and camps for prisoners of war.[24] The Canadian Red Cross managed to develop successfully at a local level. In Alberta, the Calgary Branch of the Canadian Red Cross had its first meeting in August 1914,[25] the Alberta Division in September 1914 in the office of R.B. Bennett, and the first chapter of the Junior Red Cross (for school children) was established in 1920.[26]

One of the activities of the Alberta Division of the Red Cross was caring for children who were left without parents after World War I. Children were placed in the War Orphans' Home. It was taken over by the Red Cross in 1919 from the Great War Veterans Association (GWVA)[27] and cost $4,011.21 for six months of operation. The amount of $770.87 was received as payment for board and lodging, thus the net cost to the Red Cross was $3,240.34. Salaries and rent were each over $1,000.[28]

The Alberta Division of the Red Cross also ran the Rest Home, which not only housed soldiers and their families after their return from abroad, but also some thirty-nine children whose parents could not look after them and who could not be placed in the War Orphans' Home.[29] The Rest Home closed in March 1920. Because it was not desirable to run two separate houses, the Repatriation Committee of the Alberta Red Cross Division together with the Child Welfare Committee of Calgary advised

the Red Cross Executive that a place should be found which would provide accommodation for all soldiers' children placed in the care of the
society.[30]

Large premises were needed to house so many children, and the Red
Cross looked around for grounds and a house. They did not find one
within the city but leased two houses and thirty-two acres outside the
city for $2,700 per year. Both houses were owned by E.H. Crandall and
were situated at Brickburn which was two and a half miles west of Calgary
in the Wildwood area, near a brickwork. The Soldiers' Children's Home,
or Brickburn House, opened on July 14, 1920, and had room for sixty
children.[31] It was set up primarily to care for orphans in a home-like
setting. There were also a few children who had had surgical operations
paid for by the Junior Red Cross Sick Children's Fund, a fund set up to
pay for operations for children who could not afford them. These children came from all over Alberta and parts of Saskatchewan and, following their surgery in city hospitals, went home whenever possible. Those
who could not go home were transferred to Brickburn House for convalescence. A matron was hired to supervise the medical aspects of day-to-
day life in Brickburn House.

Annual reports contain many interesting stories. In 1921, the report
tells the story of a twelve-year-old girl who came into Calgary walking on
her knees. She had walked this way for two years, with both feet pressed
tightly against the back of her upper leg. Under anaesthesia at the Calgary
General Hospital, her legs were straightened and strapped to splints, then
she went to Brickburn to convalesce. After six weeks at Brickburn, she
went home perfectly normal.

The children, whether orphans or convalescents, needed education.
As a school was not otherwise available, one was opened on the grounds.
This school was supervised and inspected by the Department of Educa-
tion and the teacher was Mabel Mappin. She taught in the Junior Red
Cross Children's Hospital once it opened.

The expenditure for Brickburn House was $28,342.23, and donations
were only $948.62, after a refund for board of $3,883.30.[32] Salaries and
wages were $11,136.35.[33] In 1921, the Society made it clear that in its
view responsibility for the care of these children was a government obligation.[34] The Red Cross therefore arranged for a government grant of
$20,000 for the care of soldiers' children in 1921. This sum was for both
the house in Calgary and the one in Edmonton. Once again, the Red
Cross stated that it would be happy to withdraw from this work should
the government take over the task.[35]

Even in 1921, there was a waiting list of over six hundred children[36]for
medical care. Assessment of all the applications for treatment were handled by an Advisory Committee of the Junior Red Cross Sick Children's
Fund. Members of this Advisory Committee were Dr. R. O'Callaghan and

Dr. R.B. Deane, who were both later connected to the Junior Red Cross Children's Hospital. Physicians in Alberta were supportive of the Junior Red Cross Sick Children's fund, and the Alberta Medical Association, at its meeting in Calgary in 1921, resolved to charge only twenty-five percent of physician fees when patients came through this fund.[37]

The Executive Committee of the Alberta Division of the Canadian Red Cross Society (January 9, 1920) asked the Child Welfare Committee to describe what was most needed and how this might tie in with the work of the Junior Red Cross. The decision to open a children's hospital was made by the Board of the Red Cross Branch on March 18, 1920, following suggestions made by the Child Welfare Committee, and one month later it was called the Children's Hospital for Alberta. A home-like setting was needed in which children could carry on their studies while convalescing. A year later, in December 1921, there were still problems: "The difficulty of procuring accommodation together with the expense involved in providing treatment for the increasing number of cases points to the necessity of steps being taken at an early date to proceed with plans for a children's hospital for the Province."[38]

On March 3, 1922, it was resolved to call it the Junior Red Cross Children's Hospital. The word "Junior" was included because it would mean a feeling of "our hospital" for the Junior Red Cross branches.[39] This would increase their interest and enthusiasm. At this point, the Junior Red Cross had already started fundraising to build a children's hospital. The members of the Junior Red Cross were innovative and often saved produce coupons as well as pennies, made coat hangers and collected used tobacco tins. The flat tobacco tins were sold to fishermen, as they were excellent for holding bait and a good fit in a hip pocket. Once money was secured, the next stage was to look for premises. An ideal location was found in a large brick building at 522 – 18 Avenue SW. The premises, previously a nursing home, were rented from a Miss Leveque.[40]

At the same time, the operation of Brickburn House was under scrutiny, and it was closed on December 31, 1922. By that time, most of the children had found other homes or were transferred to the Next-of-Kin House in Edmonton.[41] Nowadays, the former Brickburn House is a family residence.❖

References

1. *History of the Red Cross: Great Britain*. 1st ed. Lowe & Bydone, London, 1940, p. 28.
2. *The Volunteer* [a Red Cross publication], 6(1) (1955): 19.
3. Dunant, Henry. *A Memory of Solferino*. English version. Geneva, International Committee of the Red Cross, 1986, p. 2.
4. *History of the Red Cross*. p. 23.
5. Dunant, Henry. *A Memory of Solferino*. p. 106.
6. Ibid., p. 72.
7. Ibid., p. 115.

8. Ibid., p. 125.

9. *History of the Red Cross*. p. 40.

10. Ibid., p. 35.

11. Ibid., pp. 22-23.

12. Dunant, Henry. *A Memory of Solferino*. p. 132.

13. Canadian Red Cross, Southern Alberta Region, personal communication.

14. Hutchinson, John F. *Champions of Charity: War and the Rise of the Red Cross*. Westview Press, Boulder, CO, 1996.

15. Porter, McKenzie. *To All Men*. McClelland & Stewart, London, 1960, p. 29.

16. *The Volunteer*, 6(1) (1955): 1.

17. *The Volunteer*, 9(2) (1958): 4.

18. *History of the Red Cross*, p. 30.

19. "Our Red Cross Hospital," *The Canadian Red Cross Dispatch*, September 1949, p. 3.

20. *The Albertan*, February 25, 1941.

21. *History of the Red Cross*. p. 54.

22. Ibid., p. 36.

23. Ibid., pp. 57-58.

24. *Summary of Red Cross Services, Historical*. The Canadian Red Cross Society, Alberta Division, 1973, Appendix A, p. 1.

25. Lent, Geneva D. *Alberta Red Cross in Peace and War, 1914-1947 [Lent Report]*, Canadian Red Cross Society, Alberta Division, Calgary, 1947, p. 2.

26. *Calgary Branch, Alberta-Northwest Territories Division. The Canadian Red Cross Society: A Historical Account of its Development and Status as at 1976*, p. 3.

27. *Minutes*. The Canadian Red Cross Society, Alberta Division, Oct. 11, 1919.

28. *Annual Report*. Canadian Red Cross Society, Alberta Division, 1920, Schedule 51, p. 46.

29. Ibid., p. 28.

30. *Minutes*. Executive Committee, Canadian Red Cross Society, Alberta Division, March 18, 1920, p. 12. Also in *Minutes*. Repatriation Committee, Nov. 19, 1920 (Red Cross Archives).

31. *Minutes*. Executive Committee, Canadian Red Cross Society, Alberta Division, April 23, 1920.

32. *Annual Report*. Canadian Red Cross Society, Alberta Division, 1931, Exhibit, p. 40.

33. *Annual Report*. Canadian Red Cross Society, Alberta Division, 1921, Schedule 1, p. 41.

34. *Annual Report*. Canadian Red Cross Society, Alberta Division, 1921, p. 18.

35. Ibid., p. 19.

36. *Minutes*. Canadian Red Cross Society, Alberta Division, Oct. 14, 1921.

37. *Annual Report*. Canadian Red Cross Society, Alberta Division, 1921, p. 25.

38. Ibid., p. 24.

39. *Minutes*. Executive Committee, Canadian Red Cross Society, Alberta Division, March 3, 1922, p. 5.

40. Ibid., p. 6. In primary sources for the early history, names were not always given in full. In some cases, we have not been able to find the first name or initials and have cited names as found in the source.

41. *Annual Report*. Canadian Red Cross Society, 1922, p. 6.

Further reading

White, Ranald D. The Canadian Red Cross Society. Calgary Branch, 1976.

The First Junior Red Cross Children's Hospital

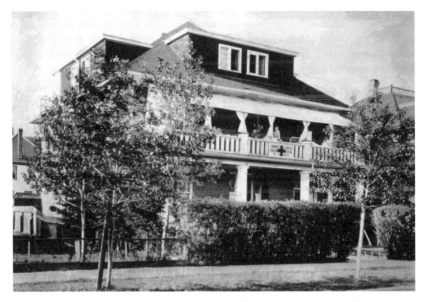

The first Junior Red Cross Children's Hospital.

The Junior Red Cross Children's Hospital, the first in Canada, was officially opened on May 19, 1922, by Lieutenant Governor R.G. Brett, himself a physician.[1] There were many other dignitaries present, including Mayor S.H. Adams and bearded Bishop Cyprian Pinkham. This hospital joined those already in existence to serve the citizens of Calgary, Canada's eighth largest city in 1922, with a population of 63,305. The first hospital was founded in 1877, as an infirmary for the Northwest Mounted Police. In 1890, the General Hospital was founded, and, in 1904, a separate wing was opened called the "Isolated Hospital." The more modern title "Isolation Hospital" was used later.[2] In 1891, the Holy Cross Hospital opened, followed by other hospitals early in the twentieth century: the Grace Hospital (1910), the Colonel Belcher (1918), and Baker Memorial Sanatorium (1920).

Some of those present at the opening of the Junior Red Cross Children's Hospital had already been actively involved in Calgary's health care. For example, Bishop Pinkham had been instrumental in starting the

General Hospital, using a legacy donated for this specific purpose by a Chinese gentleman, Jimmy Smith, who died from tuberculosis in a hotel room.[3] Moreover, Jean Pinkham, the Bishop's wife, was one of the main founders of the Women's/Ladies' Hospital Aid Society, an organization that was instrumental in the early development of the General Hospital. Finally, some young ladies had started their own society to support the Women's Hospital Aid Society. This Girls' Hospital Aid Society volunteered services and donated $700 to rent equipment when the Junior Red Cross Children's Hospital was started. The Girls' Hospital Aid Society became a Corporate Society in 1922, and its degree of involvement is clear in the statement of purpose "to relieve the physical wants and necessities of children in poor circumstances, during sickness and convalescence."[4] This organization became the Children's Hospital Aid Society (CHAS) in 1926 and still provides essential support to today's Alberta Children's Hospital.

In an advance notice, *The Albertan* announced that more than 225 invitations were sent out for the official opening ceremony of the new Children's Hospital, which would have a thirty-five-bed capacity.[5] Other reports offer some details, such as the fact that there were twenty-nine patients in the hospital on the day of the official opening.[6]

The opening itself is briefly mentioned in *The Calgary Herald* women's page, in a section called "Woman's Community Interest. Her social, club and political life."[7] The article discussed the Hospital for Sick Children in Toronto in detail and provided only limited information on Calgary's new Children's Hospital. The article the next day, however, described the purpose of the Calgary Children's Hospital: to provide free hospital care and medical treatment to children whose parents or guardians were unable to afford private care.[8] Parents who had the financial resources would more likely hire a nurse to care for the child at home or visit a doctor's office.

In his opening address, Mayor Adams proudly noted that child welfare was receiving greater attention in Calgary than in any other city in Canada. He specifically welcomed co-operation with the provincial Red Cross and assured Red Cross dignitaries that their work did not compete with the city's efforts. The precise meaning of his remark is not clear. However, at that time, there was no such thing as "a health-care system." Many organizations competed to provide health care, and the Mayor presumably had strong loyalties to the municipal hospital (Calgary General Hospital). That might also explain the fact that, in his speech, he specifically referred to the children's ward of the Calgary General Hospital. Be that as it may, Mayor Adams wholeheartedly welcomed the Junior Red Cross Children's Hospital.[9]

Even before the hospital officially opened, Claude M., a seven-year-old girl admitted with influenza, had been admitted and discharged. In the first seven days the hospital was open, eight patients were admitted. One child died a week after admission. By the end of the first month of

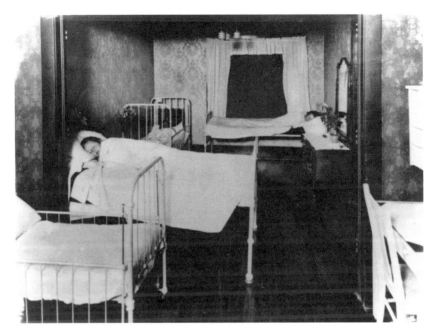

Girls' ward.

operation, eighteen children had been admitted, three died. Their ages ranged from two to sixteen years. They were admitted with a variety of diagnoses such as polio, tuberculosis, malnutrition and tonsillitis. Many stayed for weeks or months. Some of the diagnostic terms are unusual, perhaps offensive, to us, such as "congenital idiocy," which includes a range of disorders such as severe cerebral palsy, microcephaly (extremely small brain), genetic disorders and chromosomal disorders (Down Syndrome, Trisomy 21).[10] Idiocy was the lowest grade of mental defectives (another offensive label) and indicated a mental age of less than two years.[11]

The hospital was a three-storey building; girls were on the first and third floors and boys on the second floor. There was only one bathroom, on the second floor, and there was no elevator! Reports indicated that between thirty-five and thirty-eight patients could be cared for. It is likely that, in times of need, space was found for children even if the hospital was full.

The hospital, at 522 – 10 Avenue SW, was built as a duplex in 1913, both as a residence and for revenue. The owners were Joseph and Annetta Wright. Annetta Wright was a member of the Bannerman family who were prominent fur traders. The family leased the building to the Red Cross to be used as a hospital. After the Junior Red Cross Hospital moved to Lower Mount Royal, the building was remodelled into an apartment block, called the Walter Murray apartments. It stayed in the Wright family until 1950. This building is still standing.

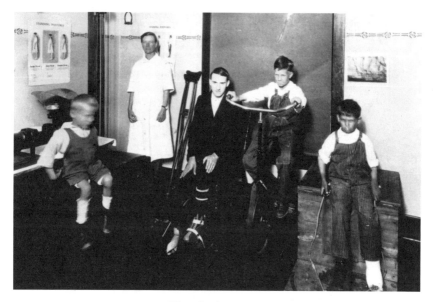

Physiotherapy.

The outside was attractive. A reporter described the appearance in the summer: "There are big window-boxes with glowing red geraniums at each of the front windows and on the veranda. All around the building are shade trees, and a carragana hedge shuts off the lawn from the street."[12] By the end of the first year of operation, 134 sick and crippled children had been admitted to the hospital; most required nursing care alone, but a few required surgery. By the fall of 1922, "The operating room is completed and minor operations are being performed."[13] Major surgery was performed either in the General or the Holy Cross hospitals. Children were transported to the Alberta Children's Hospital for post-operative care and convalescence.

Dedicated nursing care was provided by two day nurses and one night nurse supervised by Louise Peat, formerly a nurse at Mount Royal College.[14] Peat had nursed overseas with the Queen's Own British Unit of the army in Malta during the World War I. It was felt that she ran the hospital like a military operation, and, in the Red Cross *Minutes*, there were hints of discomfort at her style of management. Several charges were laid against her, but the board reached the conclusion that there had been no cruelty to children. They did feel though that there was a need for change. The matron and two nurses resigned, and Mrs. Elliott was appointed matron.[15]

A physiotherapist (Mildred Spreckley) was one of the professionals who worked with the nursing staff. Other members of staff included the cook, kitchen maid, two housekeeping maids and janitor (Mr. Pearce). All the staff members provided dedicated care and worked long hours

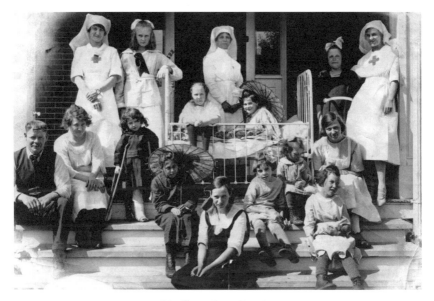

Staff and patients.

with only a few days off, and most of them remained for many years.

Some of the dedicated physicians who gave their time to the hospital were Dr. R. O'Callaghan, Dr. D.R. Dunlop, Dr. R.B. Deane, Dr. J.M. Adams (eyes, ear, nose specialist), Dr. W.H. McFarlane, Dr. E. Wright (dentist), Dr. R. Leacock (pathologist), Dr. J.L. Allen, Dr. J.N. Gunn. Six other physicians served as consultants. These physicians were volunteers. The only payment by the hospital was a salary of $100 for Dr. Deane, and the only physician to claim fees was Dr. Allen, at a quarter of the regular rate.[16]

The cost of the first Junior Red Cross Hospital was $14,680.15 per year, of which the Alberta provincial government paid $7,256. The operating cost was estimated at $1.75 per day per patient, and the provincial government partially offset this cost with one dollar per patient per day.[17] The total revenue of the Junior Red Cross Hospital from October 31, 1921, to December 31, 1922, was $10,133.53. Among numerous donors was the Girls' Hospital Aid Society, and soldiers of the 137th Battalion donated generously for the care of soldiers' children. One way of raising money was to endow a bed for a year for $200.

The Junior Red Cross Children's Hospital in Calgary provided care for children from towns and cities throughout the province. Special efforts were made to reduce travelling for children from the north, so some children had surgery at the University Hospital in Edmonton.

The Kiwanis Club of Edmonton indicated its intention to donate a Junior Red Cross Children's Home in Edmonton.[18] Thus, the Junior Red Cross Wing of the University Hospital in Edmonton was officially opened

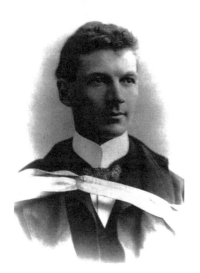

Dr. Reginald Burton Deane

F.H. Mewburn. These two doctors were raised in the West and known for their colorful and profane language.

In 1911, Dr. Deane came to Calgary and, at the age of fifty, set off for further training to enhance his skills as an orthopaedic surgeon. He returned from that training in England in 1922, joined the Alberta Children's Hospital and, until 1936, was an orthopaedic surgeon to children on a voluntary basis. The name of Dr. Deane and the Junior Red Cross Hospital have been synonymous since the opening of the hospital in 1922, where he was known for outstanding service, devotion to duty and a personal interest in the welfare of crippled children.

In addition to his activities in the operating room, he was Superintendent of the hospital, Chairman of the Board and Director of The Canadian Red Cross Society, Alberta Division.

Dr. Deane became severely ill, was given leave of absence, retired in 1939 and died in 1941.

Dr. Deane was born in England and came to Canada as a young child in 1882 with his father, R. Burton Deane, who was a Captain of the Royal Marines. His father was appointed Superintendent of the NWMP, and they were quartered in Edmonton. Dr. Deane has early memories of witnessing the hanging of Louis Riel. Eventually the family came to Calgary, and the famous Deane House was built by Captain Deane.

Dr. Deane graduated from McGill University in Medicine in 1898, registered in the Northwest Territories and practised in Maple Creek, Saskatchewan. One year later, he moved to Lethbridge and practised as an orthopaedic surgeon with Dr.

in 1927.[19] Shortly after it opened, the federal government required that building but agreed to put up a new building, which opened in 1930. Earlier, in 1925, the Regina Junior Red Cross Wing of the Regina General Hospital opened. Margaret Baxter worked in the Junior Red Cross Wing in Regina before she became Matron of the Junior Red Cross Children's Hospital in Calgary in 1952. In Regina, the staff did not feel part of the hospital, they were "over in that wing" but did not really have a separate identity. The fact that it was not a separate building may be why no children's hospital evolved from it.[20] In Calgary, the staff in the Children's Hospital "were all one."[21] ❖

References

1. Dr. R.G. Brett was one of the early physicians in the Northwest Territories and began as a Canadian Pacific Railway doctor. He ran the Hot Springs Sanatorium in Banff and was the first President of the Alberta Medical Association.
2. *Minutes*. Board of the General Hospital, Annual Reports, 1903, 1904 and 1906 in President's report.
3. Hardwick, E., E. Jameson and E. Tregillus. *The Science, the Art and the Spirit: Medicine and Nursing in Calgary*. Century, Calgary, 1975, p. 318.
4. *History of the Children's Hospital Aid Society, 1908-1979*, p. 2.
5. *The Albertan*, May 13, 1922.
6. *The Calgary Daily Herald*, May 18, 1922.
7. *The Calgary Daily Herald*, May 19, 1922.
8. *The Calgary Daily Herald*, May 20, 1922.
9. Ibid.
10. Mitchell, A.G., E.K. Upham and E.M. Wallinger. *Pediatrics and Pediatric Nursing*. W.B. Saunders & Co., Philadelphia, 1941, p. 405–409.
11. Holt, L.E., and J. Howland. *The Diseases of Infancy and Childhood*. 8th ed. D. Appleton & Co., New York, 1922, p. 766.
12. *The Red Cross Junior*. September 1922.
13. *Minutes*. Executive, Alberta Division, Canadian Red Cross Society, September 15, 1922.
14. *Minutes*. Executive, Alberta Division, Canadian Red Cross Society, March 22, 1922.
15. *Minutes*. Executive, Alberta Division, Canadian Red Cross Society, February 9, 1926.
16. *Minutes*. Executive, Alberta Division, Canadian Red Cross Society, February 23, 1923.
17. *Minutes*. Executive, Alberta Division, Canadian Red Cross Society, March 3, 1922, p. 4; May 16, 1924.
18. *Annual Report*. 1923, p. 13.
19. *Annual Report*. 1927, p. 9.
20. *Red Cross Junior*, 4(4) (1925): p. 3.
21. Margaret Baxter, personal communication.

Further reading

Jack, Donald. *Rogues, Rebels, and Geniuses: The Story of Canadian Medicine*. Doubleday, Toronto, 1981.

First Seven Years of the Children's Hospital

The future of the Junior Red Cross Children's Hospital was not at all certain when it opened in 1922. Though uncertainty comes with new ventures, usually the tone is set in the first few years. In that time, some organizations reach prominence rapidly, but then lose their apparent distinction and begin to fail. Other organizations are much slower to establish their identity with the public, but gather strength continuously and are always planning and looking to the future. Fortunately, those providing leadership to the Alberta Children's Hospital were planning even as they were dealing with the daily problems of sick and crippled children.

The Junior Red Cross Children's Hospital had three aims in its care for the crippled child. Two of the aims were obvious: achieving as much physical potential as possible and achieving a good education for the child, although this was not even attempted in many hospitals. The third aim was to offer the children occupational therapy and thus provide them with skills that could be used in later life.

The need for the hospital is shown by the steady increase in numbers throughout the 1920s. The original admission ledger has been preserved and gives an overall view of the variety of patients seen. The total number admitted between 1922 and 1929 was 792, fairly equally split between boys (402) and girls (390). The youngest child admitted was six months old and the oldest, nineteen years old, all with many different diagnoses.

Ledger of admissions

Diagnoses from 1922 to 1929

	Number	*Percentage*
Septic tonsils	152	29.9
Polio	103	20.2
Club foot	55	10.8
Osteomyelitis	52	10.2
Cerebral palsy	32	6.3
Tuberculosis	30	5.9
Malnutrition	23	4.5
Scoliosis	18	3.5
Cleft palate	16	3.1

Septic tonsils accounted for almost thirty percent of admissions and, along with polio, club foot and osteomyelitis, were responsible for more than seventy percent of admissions. The many other causes were varied and included many orthopaedic and non-orthopaedic conditions. Children stayed in the hospital for a long time by our standards, with the most common length of stay being between one and two months (median fifty-one days). Some children stayed more than one year, making the average length of stay 159 days. There had been one death in the hospital before it was opened, and by the time the first hospital closed, twenty-seven deaths had been registered. Some of the causes of death were heart disease (5), cleft lip and palate (4) and tuberculosis (3). There were other causes of death, including one child who died from the late effects of lye poisoning. Lye is a caustic alkali (sodium hydroxide and sodium hypochlorite) used for cleaning drains. At that time, it was available as granules and, when swallowed by a child, caused extensive destruction of tissues in the mouth, throat, larynx (voice box) and esophagus (gullet).[1] Such injuries are now rare in Canada but still occur in other parts of the world. The largest number of deaths in a single year was in 1922, when there were thirteen; in other years, the numbers were much smaller and, in 1927, there were no deaths. This is not of course to suggest that death in childhood did not occur anymore; rather these figures reflect the particular work of the Junior Red Cross Children's Hospital as a place for convalescence. Death in childhood was common both at home and in general hospitals.

Human stories are more interesting to most of us than statistics. Some of the stories we found are amusing, especially with a seventy-five-year perspective, some tragic and some uplifting. Many of these stories pique our interest and leave unanswered questions. For example, on November 15, 1923, three brothers and one sister were all admitted with a diagnosis of septic tonsils and were discharged eight days later. Was this an epidemic, was it the medical custom of the time or was family convenience the paramount consideration in this admission of four siblings? The precise reason for an eight-day stay for septic tonsils cannot be known with certainty, but may have had something to do with a high risk of infection at home.

One of the nurses (Dorothy Kerfoot) tells of the many outings for the children. These day trips were extremely important for the morale of children who were in hospital for such a long time. On one occasion, a number of children were taken for a boat ride on the Bow River, and one can only imagine the scene as these children were loaded and unloaded from the boat. The children were excited, having been patients in the hospital for a long time, with little opportunity to play or even to be outside. They were of many different ages, and their movements were limited by a wide variety of orthopaedic appliances. While the many volunteers and nurses were assisting in their care, the boat tipped. One of the children fell into the water. The child had a brand new body cast, which was soaking wet when she was removed from the river. The return to the hospital was fraught with anxiety, as they were unsure of their reception. Dr. Deane was certainly not impressed, but he did suggest that they let the cast dry completely. The drying in fact took many weeks, and the child remained in the cast that was so important for her treatment. When it was finally removed, maggots crawled out from under the cast.

Though the facilities were praised at the time of opening, it did not take long for some of the inadequacies of the building to become obvious. Renovations were required as early as 1923, one year after opening. The major one was enclosing the balcony on the second floor with glass. The renovations were expensive, and although many donors contributed

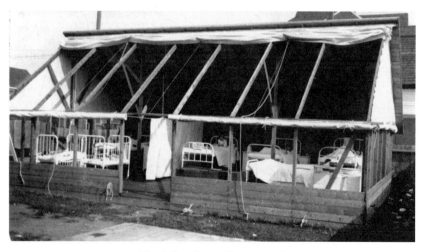

Tent for "sun therapy."

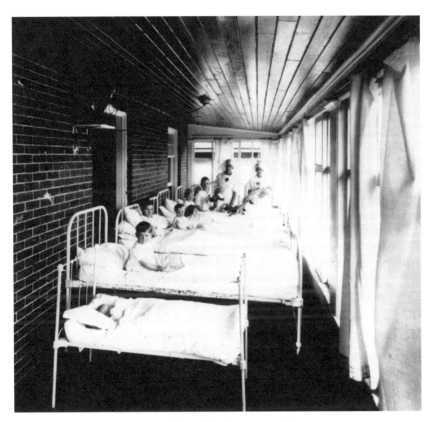

Boys' balcony.

to these renovations, the major donor for the first renovations was the Calgary Musical Club.

Heliotherapy – exposing children with tuberculosis to the sun – had become fashionable, and Dr. Deane regularly prescribed this "medical treatment." So an outside facility needed to be found, and Dr. Deane asked that a tent be erected in the back yard.[2] The Children's Hospital Aid Society raised $290.80 for this solarium, which was completed in 1925 at the back of the hospital. The tent-like structure could hold ten children at one time, half for girls and the other half for boys. Thus the summer capacity of the hospital was forty or more, but, in the winter, there were only thirty-two children at any one time.[3]

There was only one bathroom in the building at the time of opening, and children requiring its use had to be carried up and down stairs. This became even more of a problem with the development of the solarium, and accommodating more children. Therefore extensive plumbing work was carried out in the basement, and the new bathroom provided may have been the renovation sponsored by the Calgary Musical Club.

Minnie L. was a child who stayed in the hospital for a long time. Her first admission was on June 29, 1923, and was due to infantile paralysis. Although she was thirteen at the time of admission, she had to sit in a wooden stroller. By the time she left on June 30, 1925, two years had passed, but by then she was proud and happy to be walking on her own two feet. This was not the end of her contact with the Junior Red Cross Children's Hospital. She had been discharged with a corset and leg supports, which needed regular corrective work, presumably because of her growth. This was completed during her re-admission on May 11, 1926; she was in for only two weeks.

The cost of running the Junior Red Cross Children's Hospital was supported by donations. Fundraising was stimulated by the obvious need of the children. Stories about the children treated in the hospital appeared in the press and were intended to inform the public about the need for this facility. These touching stories and the subsequent publicity stimulated donations, which in turn allowed the needs of more children to be met.

Some idea of the operating cost at that time can be obtained from the report of the Junior Red Cross in 1926. A total of $10,556.35 was raised for the teatment of 169 children. Some were treated in the University Hospital in Edmonton, but most (117 of twenty different nationalities) were treated in the Children's Hospital in Calgary.[4]

The public gave generously. Many and varied gifts were not confined to money, and some were small, some large. Toys and books were given but so were fruit and vegetables. For example, three hundred jars of fruit were given in one donation.[4] All the gifts were appreciated and recorded in a book that is still available in the archives of the Alberta Children's Hospital.

The Kinsmen started a library and many of the books were donated by the Upper Canada Religious Tract and Book Society.[5] Although the hospital relied on voluntary donations for most of its operation, the government supported some activities. For example, the school, which operated for 211 days in 1926, was supported by the Department of Education which paid the salary of Mabel Mappin, the teacher. She taught regular subjects and, in addition, artificial flower-making and handicrafts.[6]

The Junior Red Cross Children's Hospital had a float in the Stampede parade, which had rapidly become popular in Calgary after its re-establishment. This float not only provided publicity, but was also a way to thank the people of Calgary for their donations and support.[7]

Near the end of the first seven years, the hospital was receiving increasing recognition locally and beginning to be recognized on a national level. In 1927, Eastern physicians are quoted as saying that the work done in this hospital in Calgary was as well done as work in Chicago or New York.[8] Of course, the statements were made in the 1927 *Annual Report* by the Commissioner of the Red Cross in Alberta, who said that he

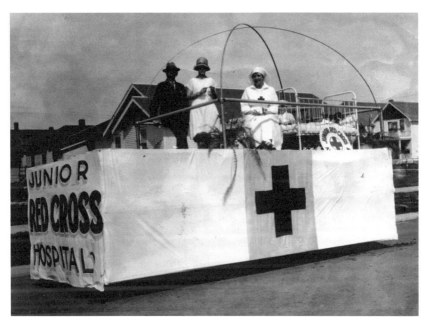

Float in Stampede parade.

had intimate knowledge of the activities at the Alberta Children's Hospital so he may not have been impartial.

Leaving the 1920s, the hospital had become well established, fulfilling a community need, and well recognized within the community. The demands on the Red Cross were increasing at this time of poverty and hardship. The same poverty reduced donations, but the Red Cross remained committed to children, particularly those whose parents could not afford treatment. In general, there were no charges, but some parents had to pay.[9] Nevertheless, the growth in the number of children served led to problems in meeting their needs. The hospital was always full, and there was a waiting list as some children remained for one to three years.

It became obvious by stages that a new hospital was needed. The idea of owning a building was more appealing to the Red Cross than continuing to pay rent, at that time $2,100 per year. The success of the institution opened in 1922 led to the opening of a new and larger hospital in 1929. The new building "occupies a very fine site in Mount Royal and has three hundred feet frontage on both streets. When the necessary alterations are made, the new building will give an immediate increased accommodation of eight beds and will have an ultimate accommodation when the top floor is finished of seventy beds. In the opinion of your Committee, the site is ideal and the removal to these new premises will make a very great advance in the work which it will be possible to carry on." [10] ❖

References

1. Arena, Jay M., ed. *Poisoning*. 5th ed. Charles C. Thomas, Springfield, IL, 1985.
2. *Minutes*. Executive Committee, Alberta Division, Canadian Red Cross Society, June 10, 1925.
3. *Annual Report*. Canadian Red Cross Society, Alberta Division, 1925, p. 57.
4. *Annual Report*. Canadian Red Cross Society, Alberta Division, 1926, p. 40.
5. Ibid.
6. *Annual Report*. Canadian Red Cross Society, Alberta Division, 1923, p. 12.
7. *The Canadian Red Cross*, 3(9) (1924): 10.
8. *Annual Report*. Canadian Red Cross Society, Alberta Division, 1927, p. 9.
9. Receipts for hospitalization of $40 in the Alberta Children's Hospital Archives.
10. *Annual Report*. Canadian Red Cross Society, Alberta Division, 1928, p. 35.

Margaret's Story

Margaret D. grew up on an Indian Reserve at Gleichen, where her father was an Anglican missionary who taught school on the reserve. She remembers that she had a Blackfoot nursemaid called Emma Big Old Man. Since she was the only one who had polio at that time on the reserve, it took a long time before the diagnosis was made.

This only came about when her mother took her to Dr. Deane in 1926. They thought she might have a "bone related disease," since her legs and feet were deformed. When Dr. Deane saw Margaret, his first exclamation was "Damn, what have you done with that child!" He was quite well known for his forceful use of language. Margaret still visualizes Dr. Deane and said that she would probably even recognize him if he walked in through the door. He was tall, skinny with glasses and a large Roman nose. He did not have much hair. Periodically, he would visit the children in the hospital, but his office was in the Grain Exchange building on 1st Street and 9th Avenue.

Margaret was a patient from 1928 to 1931. She was admitted when she was six years old with infantile paralysis. She remembers the hospital as a small house, with two girls to a room. Her room-mate was also a polio patient.

The matron of the hospital was strict and authoritarian; none of the children would even dream of not listening to or disobeying her.

In 1929, all the patients moved to the new building. This house was quite a lot larger than the first one, and now all of a sudden, they were placed in a ward. They were also able to enjoy the large gardens around the hospital, and there used to be a gardener who loved children and would compare the girls to the flowers he had just planted. They especially liked to be compared to daffodils! If they were a bit more daring, they could slide down the fire chutes from the second floor, trying not to get caught.

During a diphtheria epidemic, all the patients had to go to the Isolation Hospital, a branch of the General Hospital, and get their shots there. After that they were in quarantine. That coincided with one of the few visits that Margaret would have from her parents, because they lived so far away on the reserve. Her parents could not come in and actually talk to their child. They had to stay outside and visit through a window. She ended up seeing them two or three times in the two and a half years that she was in the hospital. Looking back, she said that it took her quite a while to re-establish contact with her parents.

The stay in the hospital was very much like being at home, especially with so many volunteers who came in to treat the kids. Birthday parties organized by the Kinsmen, for example, were celebrated in the solarium, actually a tent. These gentlemen would also take three or four children on car rides and buy big ice cream cones for a nickel at the Model Dairy on Second Street. Another big hit, of course, was the Stampede. There was not as much variety as today because, back in the early thirties, the main attraction was the stock. The kids would see cows and cows and bulls and more prize bulls from the grandstand. After that they would be treated to sandwiches and cookies in the Red Cross Hut. This space was shared with a large number of lost children who were taken care of there.

Obviously, there were quite a few patients who needed braces, and there was no brace maker in the hospital yet, so the Kinsmen would bring a couple of patients down to a little shop near the old General Hospital. The owner took pride in his work and made sure that the braces were just right. Margaret also had a night boot that was strapped on every evening, and the heavy metal brace for her leg was fixed to the boot and then tied around her leg with straps. During the day, she got a lot of practice from all kinds of exercises that the physiotherapist, Mildred Spreckley, had devised. There was a wooden apparatus where she had to pull ropes to strengthen her legs.

All her practice paid off after about two years, when she was finally discharged. After regular visits to the out-patient clinic, she was admitted again in 1940, when she was operated on by Dr. Townsend in the General Hospital. This was quite successful and after spending two months in the hospital, she was able to participate in the enjoyments of teenage life, such as skating and dancing. She still went to see Mildred Spreckley for tea at her apartment by the firehall. Although the dedicated physiotherapist was retired, she always had energy for an hour-long leg massage. They would reminisce about the years Margaret spent in the Alberta Children's Hospital, and, inevitably, the many hours that Miss Spreckley read to the children in bed would come up. This used to be so relaxing that they always fell asleep.

PART THREE

THE SECOND HOSPITAL
1929–1952

❖❖❖❖❖❖❖❖❖❖❖❖❖

Opening of the Second Children's Hospital

O n July 23, 1929, a group of excited children, among them Annie Z., a five-year-old spastic paraplegic, moved from the old hospital to the new building in Mount Royal.[1] Annie had been admitted to the old hospital in 1927 and was discharged from the new hospital in 1931. Her eyes must have widened when she saw the beautiful wards and so much more space than she had been used to in her two years in hospital. For her, this new hospital must have truly seemed the "the house

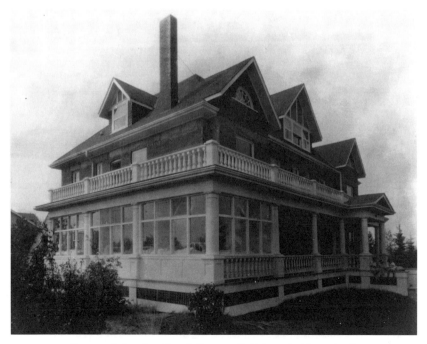

Second Junior Red Cross Children's Hospital.

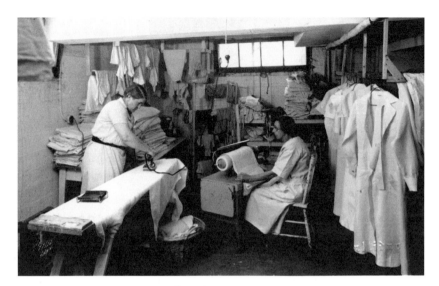

Ironing room.

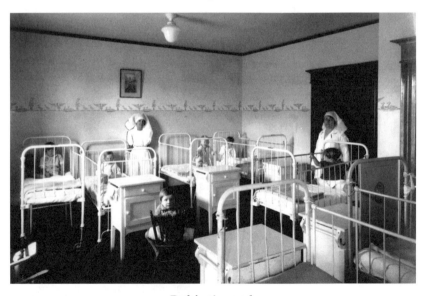

Babies' ward.

of happiness on the hill."[2] The renovated building, now owned by the Red Cross, was spacious with many wards, an operating room, a gymnasium, schoolroom, sewing room on the third floor, better accommodation for nurses right on the premises and a laundry room in the basement. The Red Cross itself moved its offices from downtown to the new hospital. The formal opening came later, on September 16, 1929.[3]

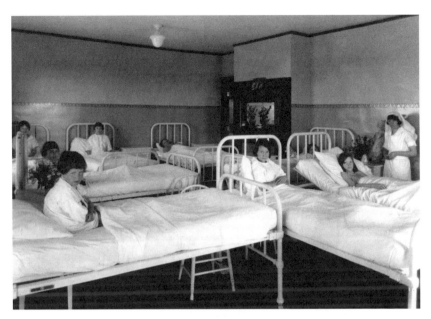

Girls' ward.

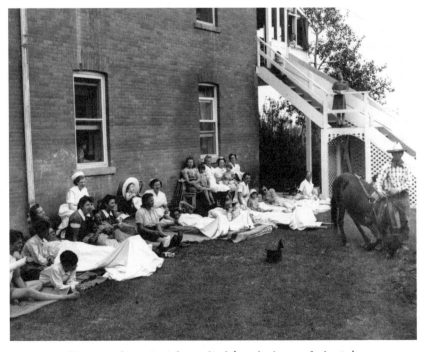

Stampede act at hospital (and view of chute).

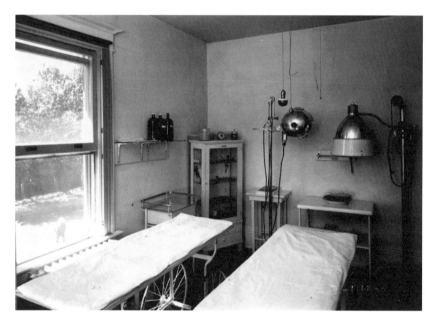

Operating room for minor operations, also doubled as heliotherapy treatment room.

The new building used to be an apartment block on 20th Avenue (1009 Royal Avenue SW) called the Ruby Apartments. This house had been built around 1911 by the architect Phileas Laurendeau, with his family living on the first floor and his sister Virginia Ruby and her family on the second floor. These families left their home about 1920.[4] According to the Red Cross Report, in 1929, R.B. Bennett was the owner of the house, which he donated to the Red Cross,[5] but other records suggest that R.B. Bennett donated a substantial amount of money to buy the house.

The new hospital, which could accommodate up to forty patients, was to be more than just a hospital though; it was also to be a home for the children. The wards were spacious and colorful. There was a Nursery funded by the Samaritan Club. The small children had a ward decorated in pale blue, with a nursery border of Peter Pan and his friends. The older boys and girls had separate wards in old ivory and primrose, and in all the wards, blue, ivory and primrose were the colors of curtains and the bedspreads. The Girls' Ward on the second floor included a pavilion, but even more interesting was a large metal (aluminum) chute at the southwest end of that floor. Its official designation was "Fire Escape," but what an exciting place to slide down if a child was quick and unobserved.[6] The Boys' Ward faced south and their balcony was called the "Sun Ward." This balcony had special glass (Vita glass) which was thought to have healing powers. The glass had been donated by the Pilkington Glass

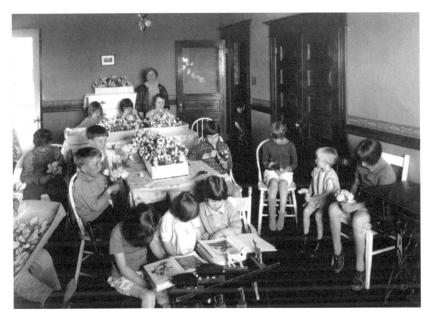

Schoolroom.

Company.[7] The children loved lying on the balcony with the light coming in, and they felt as if they were out on the lawn in the open air. They were also able to see twinkling city lights at night. In the winter, this balcony had some drawbacks. The only heating was a gas stove, and when the weather became severe, the nurses had to wear sweaters and overshoes, not to mention how cold the patients must have been. This changed in 1937 when, following a donation by the Calgary Rotary Club co-ordinated by a father of one of the patients, plumbing was installed and the ward heated.[8]

The nurses had duties in more than one ward.[9] Nurses in the Boys' Ward were responsible for the toilet room, the service entry and maintaining supplies. Those in the Infant Nursery had to take care of the diet kitchen and any adult patients. These adult patients were in fact their own colleagues. Staff members were admitted because of illnesses such as influenza or for procedures such as tonsillectomy. This practice of admitting adults occurred only during the time Florence Reid was Matron (1933-52). This may have been because of financial pressures. In the fall of 1933, lack of funding led to a reduction from fifty to twenty-five beds for patients and closure of the Nurses' Quarters.[10] The nurses in the Girls' Ward were responsible for helping in the operating room. They would set up for surgical procedures, assist the surgeons during the procedures and clean up afterwards.

The Night Nurse had to make sure doors were locked at 7 p.m., mainly because by that time drug addicts entered the hospital looking for opiates.

The operating room itself, although small, was compact, a bright spectacle of shining enamel. The operations performed varied, but in 1946 there were forty-six operations. Twenty were tonsils and adenoids and others included tendon transfers, cutting the Achilles tendon, reduction of fractures and skin grafts. In addition, over ninety casts were applied.

After operations and treatments, Mildred Spreckley, a registered nurse who had trained in physiotherapy at St. Thomas Hospital, London, England, would work with the children in the new gymnasium. Here the children learned to use their limbs once more. If not in physiotherapy, the children were in school. Mabel Mappin carried on both regular school education and occupational education until 1932 when she was succeeded by Mrs. Cotterell.[11] As part of their occupational education, the children still made artificial flowers, which were ordered from all over the world, as far as Japan and Scotland. While working with the flowers, they listened to radio, by now well established, since there were loudspeakers in every ward, connected to a central area. The Kinsmen donated the radio system in the hospital.

The new hospital also required some new equipment. For example, the Kinsmen had donated a quartz lamp for creating artificial sunlight. This light was called an Alpine Lamp, and the rules surrounding use of this valuable lamp were strict. It should not be dusted by a maid, but could only be cleaned by one particular nurse who received special training in the care of the lamp. If the lamp was touched by a finger, the mark remained, so that the required cleaning was with absolute alcohol, gauze or silk, and the nurse wore gloves.[12] Later, in 1939, the quartz lamp was replaced by another (the Hanover Quartz Lamp) at a cost of $375. The quartz (mercury vapor) lamps produced artificial sunlight, but the lamps varied in efficiency and deteriorated after a number of hours of use. They were standardized and their performances were checked regularly.

As mentioned earlier, the Red Cross was the owner of the building, and most of the costs came from the general funds of the Red Cross, although a bank loan of $8,300 was required for part of the total cost of $20,000. This loan was backed by Senator Pat Burns. There were also specific donations. The Samaritan Ward was furnished by the Samaritan Club. The Children's Hospital Aid Society remained active and supportive of the Children's Hospital, donating an eight-bed ward in memory of Edythe Lilley at a cost of $2,000 per year. She was remembered as a tireless advocate of the Junior Red Cross Children's Hospital. Many citizens donated funds for beds, and their names were inscribed on a brass plate on the end of the bed. Sometimes more than one plaque was attributed to a specific bed or a specific ward. If a particular donor was due to visit the hospital, the required plaque would be removed from storage.

The one on the bed, perhaps honoring another donor, would be quickly removed, and the appropriate plaque placed in position.❖

References

1. *Annual Report*. Canadian Red Cross Society, Alberta Division, 1929, p. 13.
2. *The Calgary Daily Herald*, June 7, 1930, p. 27.
3. *The Calgary Daily Herald*, September 14, 1929.
4. G. Christensen, personal communication.
5. *Summary of Red Cross Services*. Canadian Red Cross Society, Alberta Branch, 1973, Appendix 4A, p. 2.
6. F. McClure, personal communication.
7. *The Calgary Daily Herald*, June 7, 1930, p. 27.
8. *Annual Report*. Canadian Red Cross Society, Alberta Division, 1927, p. 5.
9. *Nursing Procedures Book*, Alberta Children's Hospital (undated, probably late 1920s or early 1930s).
10. *Annual Report*. Canadian Red Cross Society, Alberta Division, 1933, p. 19.
11. *Annual Report*. Canadian Red Cross Society, Alberta Division, 1932.
12. Gamgee, K.M.L. *The Artificial Light Treatment of Children in Rickets, Anaemia, and Malnutrition*. H.K. Lewis & Co., London, 1927, p. 63.

Patients' Experiences

The many children who came to the Junior Red Cross Children's Hospital must have had mixed feelings. They were separated from their family, lonely and scared, sometimes did not speak the language, yet they experienced and welcomed the love and care of the staff and definitely appreciated the improvement in their condition when they went home.

The Red Cross did its utmost to offer the best possible treatment to children.[1] For example, in 1931, one boy was struck on the nose with a baseball, and the injury developed into osteomyelitis. Surgeons in Calgary suggested that this boy go to Toronto for attention by a plastic surgeon. The Ontario Junior Red Cross made this possible, and the boy travelled across Canada to receive care in Toronto.[2] Even today, when air travel is commonplace, this is a long trip for a child. The trip at that time was by rail and would have been both frightening and exciting, as few children made the trip from Calgary to Toronto. Many immigrants would have come in the reverse direction, but with little expectation that they would ever leave Calgary again on such a long trip. Thus, the experience would make this boy quite different from his friends. On the long trip, he was supervised and helped by train officials along the way. At each stop, he was met by representatives of the Red Cross to check whether he was okay. Once in Toronto, the infection in his nose healed well with appropriate treatment, and he returned to Calgary cured.

While it was unusual for children to travel far away from Calgary for treatment, many of the patients of the Junior Red Cross Children's Hospital came from long distances to get the best possible care. One father, a dirt farmer from a town on the U.S. border, came only to find that the hospital was filled and could not admit his baby. The father was so convinced that the Red Cross Hospital would help his child, that he saw Colonel D.L. Tomlinson, Red Cross Commissioner, in Calgary. Because of the father's conviction, the child was placed in the isolation ward until a bed became available. There were other stories of patients and families travelling long distances. For example, a young nurse from a mission at Wabasca travelled for three nights and four days to get from her mission to the Junior Red Cross Children's Hospital. She brought two Native boys, Moise who was four years old and had previously been in hospital with club feet and congenital heart disease and Stanley, who had tuberculosis of the bones.[3]

Also a father wrote to Florence Reid, the Matron, that his seven-year-old son had just won a race event. This child had had club feet and had been admitted to the hospital at the age of one year. At that time, his feet were so badly turned in that he was totally unable to stand. He had two operations and stayed in the hospital for five months.[4] The proud moment which crowned his progress came several years later.

Juliette was a patient on many different occasions in the late 1930s. Her longest admission was two and a half years, and she saw her father only once in that time period as he had to travel from their home village, 230 kilometres northeast of Edmonton, and did not see her mother or her siblings. She clearly remembers that at the time of her first admission, she was fluent in French, and her father taught her two words of English just before he left her. By the time she returned home, she was fluent in English and could barely remember French. She came from a Roman Catholic family, but had learned all the Protestant hymns from the Sunday hymn singing. Florence Reid, the Matron, led hymns every Sunday evening for one hour; one week it was from the Boys' Ward, the next week from the Girls' Ward, each time over the intercom.

Juliette spent so much time in hospital that she was virtually raised by the nurses, which made her quite different from her siblings. She feels that she was much more independent, which gave her many advantages in life. The excellent schooling she received in hospital laid the ground work for further education. At first, she had to lie flat, and the teacher came to her, but she was always ready. Her school work was in a bag adorned with a red cross that hung on the end of her bed.

Every time Juliette was discharged home, her sisters were waiting anxiously for her, or perhaps for the presents! Juliette, like every child discharged from the hospital, was given a box full of toys and books, and beautiful dolls with eyes that would open and close. It did not matter that she was in hospital many different times, she was given a present each time.

Doreen was admitted in 1946 at the age of seven years with Still's disease, and she stayed for three years. Still's disease was described by an English paediatrician, G.F. Still, and is the childhood counterpart of rheumatoid arthritis in adults. There are many different forms, and many children have a good outcome. She was treated with weights and pulleys to prevent her joints, and therefore her limbs, from taking unnatural positions as they contracted. While Doreen was in hospital, her ten-year-old sister Helen was admitted in 1948 with a slipped epiphysis. The epiphysis is at the end of the bone, the part at which growth occurs. This sometimes slips in children approaching adolescence and generally heals with a long period of rest. Helen's treatment was to be put in a leg frame with a ten-pound weight and to stay in traction until discharged, thirteen months later. The sisters were not allowed to share a room, as each room was divided into age groups, and the rooms had between two and four patients. Doreen, the younger sister, was in a room with a girl who had been badly burnt in a grass fire. This girl was in so much pain and distress that she had to be removed. Although they were in such a small hospital a long time, the sisters hardly saw one another. Sometimes on Sundays their paths would cross as they were taken to the same religious service.[5]

Both girls remembered many activities, but the highlight was undoubtedly their parents' visit. Visiting hours described in the *Nursing Procedures Book*, were from 2:30 to 3:30 p.m. for city people on Wednesdays and weekends. Their mother came on Wednesday, and their father came on Sunday. Siblings were not allowed to visit, and in the three years Doreen was in hospital, she saw her new baby brother only once. She was dressed up for the special occasion and taken to the balcony to look down at her little brother who was standing in the street. He was looking up at the sister he had never seen before and would only begin to know once she was discharged.

Visitors would bring presents for the children, but any presents of food (and that really means candy) had to be left in the Matron's office. She saved it until Saturday (called candy day), when the candy was shared among all the children. There were many ways to get around the rules, and in Doreen's case, her father used items for her doll's house as an excuse. For example, he would bring an oven, and put a small candy inside.

The pace of the hospital was slow, and all of the children knew that they would be there for a long time. Dr. Townsend saw them perhaps only once per month, but the children regarded him as a God-like figure. He would look briefly at them, look at the chart, and then say "Well this looks good, I will see you next month." For children with complicated problems, there would be discussion at orthopaedic rounds, which Doreen remembers quite well.

The nurses compensated for the lack of contact with parents and grew close to the children; to a great extent, they were substitute parents. They were with the children as they did their school work and supported them every step on the way to recovery. Nurses were very proud when "their children" left the hospital walking. To illustrate how close the relation could be, Doreen exchanged cards every Christmas with one of the nurses until 1990.

Even though the nurses were supportive, the regime was strict. The children were basically spoon fed, and Doreen, who spent a long time in hospital, vowed never to eat or even touch beets or sardines again after she left the hospital. The *Nursing Procedures Book* states that children are not required to finish everything on their plates, but are asked to eat some of everything (about half) so that their diet will remain balanced. There were sanctions. When an article of food in the main course was left untouched by a child on a general diet, dessert was withheld. There were some foods that children did not have to eat, and this odd collection of foods included raw onion, cocoa and ice cream! Candies were only given to children over two years of age, and as far as ice cream was concerned, only children who had reached the age of three were allowed this treat. School work was an integral part of the hospital routine. Both sisters remember doing school work for four or five hours every day as soon as they were dressed and had their breakfast. They had a correspondence course and were able to continue their regular grades. The education was so good that, once discharged from the hospital, they were able to return to their former school and had no problems in being integrated with their old friends or the school work. This integration was a little easier for Helen who had been away for one year, and when she returned to school with a brace, the other children were curious about it. She took this curiosity in her stride and continued with her school life and social life.

These sisters have many more fond memories, including the Christmas party given by the Kinsmen, who gave up their own Christmas morning to be with children in the hospital. Once Helen was discharged, she was able to listen to her sister Doreen on the radio, sending a message to the rest of the family.

At the same time as Doreen, "Tim" was in hospital. He had contracted tuberculosis as a child.[6] His tuberculosis progressed to affect his hips, and he was unable to walk. He was bandaged and strapped into a frame which stayed on for so long that

Tim accepted it as part of his body. Moreover, he was not the only one with a frame, there were many children who looked just like him. In the Junior Red Cross Children's Hospital, he was also offered good nutrition, rest, sunshine and play. These, perhaps as much as the specific treatments, allowed his body and mind to develop. Tim entered classes in the hospital as soon as possible. Later the frame was discarded, and he was able to join in childhood games rather than just watch. He was five and a half years old before he could sit on the side of his bed and swing his feet. Imagine his joy when he had to go downtown to have his first pair of boots made. It is no surprise that he was so excited that he went to sleep in them. Because his hip joint had not healed enough to bear his weight, he needed a special caliper and further training and instructions before he could walk. This was mastered in record time; he had decided that he was going to leave on crutches rather than with a walker. After he had been discharged, he had to visit the Out-patient Department many times until his hip was big enough to undergo surgery and could be corrected to bear his weight. He was looking forward to the surgery, because after he would be able to walk.

References

1. *The Calgary Daily Herald*, January 16, 1932.
2. *Canadian Red Cross Junior*, 11(4) (Toronto, April 1932): 2.
3. *The Calgary Herald*, April 29, 1939, p. 23.
4. Ibid.
5. *Nurses' Procedures Book*, p. 102.
6. "Human Interest in an Orthopaedic Hospital." Transcript prepared for Clare Wallace's radio broadcast, April, 1946.

Success and Growth

The new hospital in the former Ruby Apartments was operational from 1929 to 1952, during which period there were 2,523 admissions and many more children seen at the out-patient clinic. The Red Cross ran the hospital, and the costs were largely met by voluntary donations.

The children treated came from all parts of Alberta. In 1931, for example, about three quarters of the children came from rural communities, most likely reflecting the population distribution of Alberta at that time. Preference was given to children of soldiers and those whose parents could not afford medical treatment. The conditions treated (in the hospital) were mainly orthopaedic, such as infantile paralysis, tuberculosis of the bones, congenital dislocation of the hips, club feet, osteomyelitis, spinal curvature and many different kinds of fractures. In 1933, the policy of admitting just orthopaedic cases was formally adopted.[1]

The out-patient clinic was officially registered as a department in 1935.[2] Margaret Parker was in charge, described by Dr. Townsend as "a nurse with a great deal of charm, and the ability to extract maximum effort from people in order to accomplish a job."[3] The graph gives some idea of

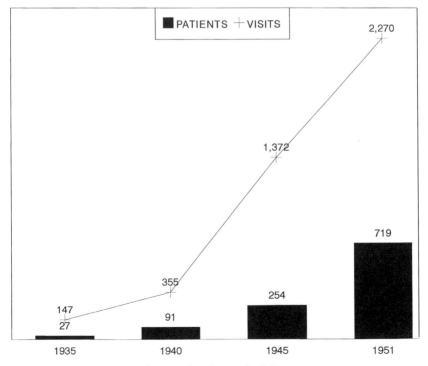

Out-patients and visits.

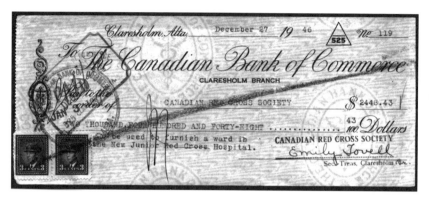

Donation, 1946.

the growth in the work of this department. The orthopaedic surgeon who ran the clinic every Thursday morning until about 2 p.m. examined children, who were fitted with appliances and returned for massage and exercise. Many children with club feet were treated entirely as out-patients, and thus the DAT concept was really an extension of an old concept, rather than a brand new idea of the 1970s.[4] Full recovery demanded attention to the proper nutrition of the children, as well as the technical aspects of their orthopaedic care. There is no doubt that many of these children were poor and malnourished.

Funds were still an issue, but the government paid some of the cost. The Junior Red Cross members were still raising money by many different methods which included collecting and selling gopher tails and magpie and crow eggs. These funds were used to buy personal items for the children as well as to defray some of the cost of running the hospital.

The library in the new hospital had over a thousand books. These were available to the children while in hospital, and once they went home each child was given five books. Some of the children had many admissions, and they were never disappointed. Each time they were discharged, they were given another five books.[5] Every year, more than five hundred books were sent home with children.

The book list is no longer in existence but many children's books were available then, some with a Canadian theme. Some were already old, such as the Christian moralizing adventure *A Tale of the Rice Lake Plains* (C.P. Traill, 1851) or the animal story *The Kindred of the Wild* (C.G.D. Roberts, 1902). The still popular *Anne of Green Gables* by L.M. Montgomery was first published in 1908. Other animal and adventure stories were new, such as *The Life of an Atlantic Salmon* (R. Haig-Brown, 1931) and *The Adventures of Sajo and her Beaver People* (Grey Owl, 1935). There were many popular books for children written in other countries, but with general appeal that were available to the children at the Alberta

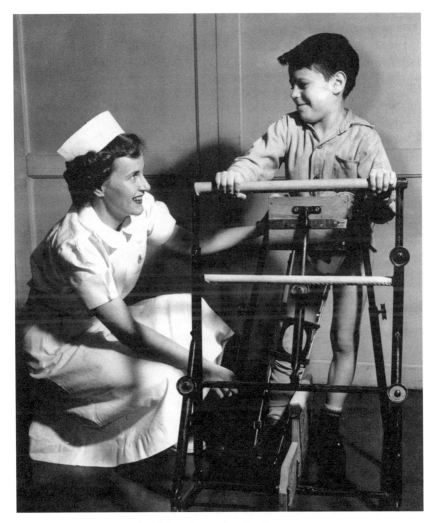

Child having physiotherapy.

Children's Hospital in the 1930s and 1940s and are still enjoyed today. These range from *Alice in Wonderland* (Lewis Carroll, 1886) to *The Tale of Peter Rabbit* (Beatrix Potter, 1901) and *Pinocchio* (Carlo Collodi, 1927).

The gymnasium on the third floor was a major feature of the hospital, and the activities were led, as mentioned earlier, by Mildred Spreckley. Exercises were for all of the patients, no matter how young. For example, Leona L., who was only eighteen months old and recovering from polio, had to practise exercises, which included grabbing the nurse's finger to regain the strength in her hand.[6] One older boy remembers being "hoisted in a sling" up the stairs to go to his physiotherapy exercise.[7] The

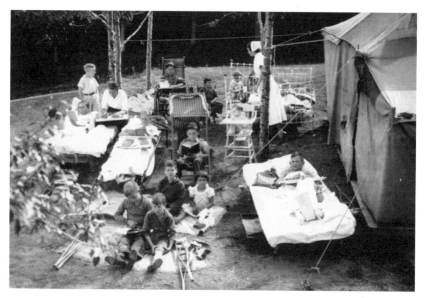

Summer at the hospital.

physiotherapist supervised the exercises, and the nurses were given specific training in physiotherapy so the treatment could be carried on even when the physiotherapist was away.

Children who could leave their beds were able to go to the open-air balconies and "in Calgary's mild climate, many of the patients are able to sleep outside the entire year."[8] Only a few patients at a time could do this, but they could enjoy the splendid view of Calgary. To allow all children the benefit of sun and fresh air, funds were donated by the Rotary Club for a new solarium large enough for eight beds which was built in 1938,[9] and not only the children slept outside, but the Matron, Florence Reid, would sleep in her little tent outside all summer long.[10]

Nursing duties were broad, in contrast to the more circumscribed role of the librarian or the physiotherapist. Nurses were given specific training for many of the different tasks of the hospital. There was also teaching for the nurses in the care of the children. Nurses who were training at the Provincial Nursing Aide School in southern Alberta attended the Alberta Children's Hospital for some of their practicum. The permanent nursing staff had a high level of expertise, so that when the nurses left, there was a gap until someone else could be trained in the specialized work done in the hospital. In those days, nurses always left when they got married, and from time to time, some nurses moved away to other hospitals.

Quite a few staff members were devoted to the hospital and stayed for a long time. A wonderful example is the Mather family. James Mather

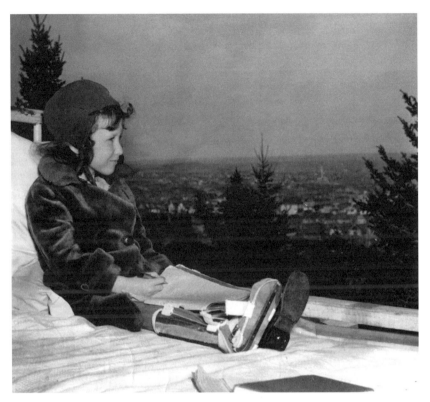

Outside, looking over Calgary.

started as a janitor in 1927 and stayed for thirty-five years. He became interested in making splints, and later devoted all of his time to this task. He worked in the specially designed brace shop, and Dr. Deane helped by giving specific descriptions of the braces required. James Mather was joined by his son, James Junior, who wanted further training and went to Toronto in 1947 for a course paid for by the Department of Veterans' Affairs[11] to study new developments in prosthetics. On returning to Calgary, his newly gained knowledge was immediately put to use. Artificial limbs were his specialty. They were made out of willow blocks that had been dried for seven years and were both strong and lightweight. Stretched rawhide was used for substitute skin, and flesh-colored paint made the limb almost lifelike. James also made all the difficult braces, such as those for scoliosis. To remain up to date, James returned to Toronto in 1957, paid for by the CHAS, to take training in plastic protheses, although even then wood was used if children had allergies. Another son, Jack, also joined the family workshop and was the steam engineer. He worked as a bootmaker until a qualified person was hired. He then helped out in brace making. The Alberta Red Cross Crippled Children's Hospital was

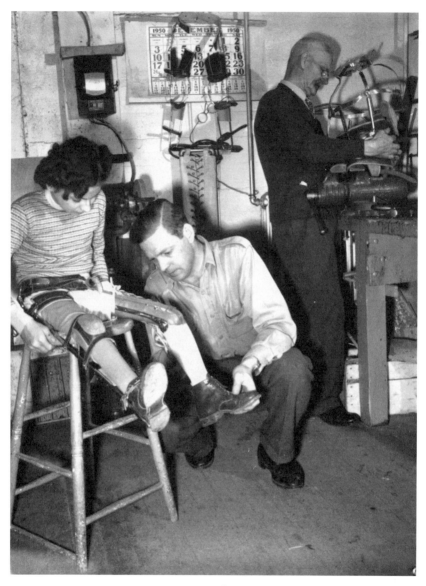

Brace shop.

one of the few hospitals in Canada that had its own brace shop and made its own artificial limbs.

The medical staff continued to volunteer their services. Dr. R.B. Deane was Medical Superintendent; his associates included Dr. F.T. Campbell, Dr. M.G. Cody, and Dr. J.W. Auld. Dr. R. O'Callaghan, who had been in the first hospital, left Calgary in 1932. Dr. Deane resigned from the staff

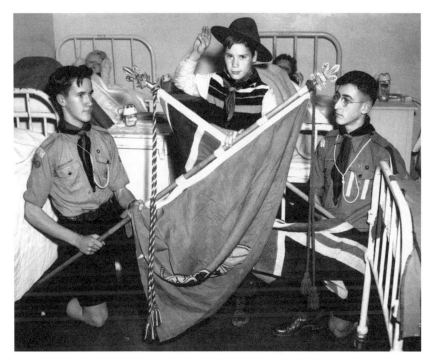

Scouts.

of the hospital on December 31, 1939, due to ill health. Dr. Campbell was appointed Medical Superintendent and Orthopaedic Surgeon, and, at that time, Dr. Gordon Townsend and Dr. E.A. Selby joined the staff. Dr. Townsend had just started practice in Calgary as a trained orthopaedic surgeon and supervised the poliomyelitis patients who were treated under the *Poliomyelitis Sufferers' Act*. These physicians always entered the hospital through the back door and kitchen to avoid climbing the front stairs.

Volunteers remained an essential part of the hospital. There were between two and three hundred volunteers who gave direct service to the hospital and many others who volunteered as fundraisers. Many volunteers approached the hospital directly, as they wished to work in the hospital with the children, other volunteers were members of organizations such as Kinsmen or the Red Cross and came to the hospital under the aegis of the other organization. All of this help ensured that there was an activity for the children every night of the week. On Monday evening, trained librarians came in, Tuesday, the Girl Guides, Wednesday evening, singers from a choral group, Thursday, Boy Scouts, Friday, a play group for older children. Every night bedtime stories were read to the younger children. Whenever a child had a birthday, girls from Western Canadian High School provided birthday cakes and a present.[12] Members of the

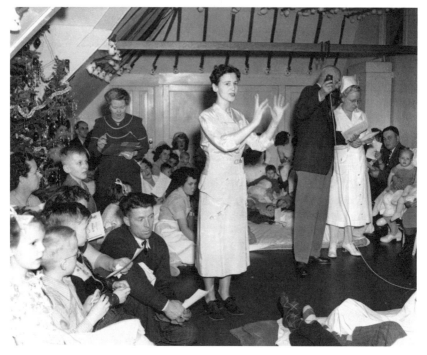

Christmas party.

Kinsmen Club arrived on Saturday afternoon in their cars to take patients who could be moved for a drive and an ice cream. Other patients went to a picture show put on by the Kinsmen, usually old cowboy films. Crafts were also supervised by volunteers, and everyone from this era of the hospital remembers Walter Ricks from the Canadian National Institute for the Blind (CNIB), himself blind, who taught basket weaving.[13] They used to say: "If Mr. Ricks can be so particular about our work and he can't even see then we should be particular too."[14]

There were hardly any visitors, so the many activities were important. Children from far away hardly saw their family and, to ease the financial strain, the Junior Chamber of Commerce supplied funds for transportation and accommodation of parents who had no money to pay for it themselves. This lasted well into the 1950s.

Volunteers participated heavily in the major annual events at Stampede and Christmas. Patients who were fit enough to be moved would be brought to the Grandstand on flatbeds and put directly onto cars. At Christmas time, a tree was donated by the Kinsmen Club and decorated profusely with lights. The tree was placed in the school room. Every child in the hospital was carried up there to receive presents from Santa Claus. The whole party was broadcast live on radio, and each child sent greetings to parents and family at home. Although this radio show was made possible by the efforts of volunteers, it was hard for parents and children not to be together.

The Kinsmen were active in helping the children and organized an outing to see the King and Queen as an extra special treat in 1939. The thrill of that visit would be similar to the visit of a sports hero or pop star today. A special site was chosen and prepared to give a clear view of the spectacle, one of the many details that helped to make this a memorable experience for the children.

Finances remained a concern throughout the 1930s and 1940s. In some of the Depression years, two wards were closed for the summer to reduce expenses, and wages were cut. In 1930, a senior graduate nurse received $80 per month, plus room and board, and this was certainly considered a good wage. However, by 1933, the three senior nurses had their wages halved to $40 per month, and the two junior nurses were given even less at $25 per month. There was an third junior nurse who had the choice of leaving the hospital or becoming a kitchen aid. She chose to stay in the hospital as a kitchen aid, receiving only $15 per month.[15] Salaries remained the main expenditure; for example, in 1935, the amount spent on salaries for the running of the hospital was $7,251.26, which paid for a number of members of staff including a matron, nurses, physiotherapist, cook, two maids and a janitor. The teacher was paid by the Board of Education.

The nurses were asked to economize; it was believed that there was a widespread tendency "to fail to appreciate the value of things when they are financed by an institution and not by oneself. If each member of the staff will feel it her particular concern to avoid waste, funds can be used to a much fuller service."[16]

However, donations kept coming in and were supplemented by government grants for special groups such as polio patients. As before, the gifts were not only money, but also in kind such as flour, groceries, eggs (delivered to the back door of the hospital). These were all duly noted in the donation book, and the gifts of fresh food were prepared for the children as soon as possible. Canada Flour Mills donated enough flour and cereals for a whole year.

The Alberta Children's Hospital still concentrated on orthopaedic cases and did not participate in care of the acutely ill, who were admitted to the Calgary General Hospital or Holy Cross Hospital or were looked after at home. There were major changes overall in childhood diseases, with less severe infectious diseases and fewer deaths. Death in childhood was now less common, and the most common age of death for children was in the first four weeks of life. One index of this change and improvement is the infant death rate, which fell from 92.9/1,000 in 1929 to 38.5/1,000 by 1951.

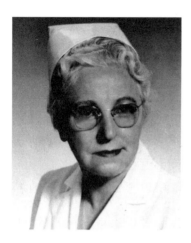

Florence Reid

at the University of Alberta in administrative nursing. She became Director of Public Relations and Welfare in 1952 and remained in that position until her retirement in 1962. She was responsible for many programs that grew with the development of the hospital, but it was always important to her that there should be a home-like atmosphere. It was well recognized that the children loved her.

She was given many honors, including the King George V Jubilee decoration in 1935 for her "outstanding contribution to nursing in the field of the public health" and was elected "outstanding citizen of the year" by the Junior Chamber of Commerce in 1952 with a citation that read "For untiring work on behalf of many children." In 1961, she received a testimonial plaque from the Alberta Children's Hospital.

She died August 10, 1981, and was described as very soft-spoken, with a wonderful personality. She was always dedicated to her work and to the care of children and had a strong rapport with children and with their parents.

Florence Reid came west with her parents from Ontario as a young girl and spent two years with the United Church Mission while she worked in a children's shelter. During the First World War, her fiancé, Percy Young, was killed and that event affected the course of her life. She trained as a nurse at the Archer Memorial Hospital in Lamont, Alberta, graduated in 1924 and immediately afterwards taught public health at the Vermilion Agriculture College and did district nursing in the Hanna and Peace River area. By 1932, she was named Field Organizer and Nursing Supervisor for the Alberta Division of the Canadian Red Cross Society.

In May 1933, she was appointed Matron of the Junior Red Cross Children's Hospital. She took a course

The Red Cross, and all of the professionals involved, looked at the work of the hospital and the need for a new hospital and started a building fund (in the 1940s). An increase in accommodation was thought necessary because there was a long waiting list. In 1942, there were forty-four patients on the list,[17] and some had to wait up to two years. The waiting list for the Junior Red Cross Crippled Children's Hospital was one measure of need, but looking more widely, Dr. M. Cody estimated that in 1947, there were over 1,600 crippled children in Alberta. The Red Cross started looking at a variety of sites, including an eight-acre location between the Glencoe Club and Earl Grey Public School. The site that was eventually used for the new building was identified by the end of the war, between 19th and 21st Streets and 17th and 19th Avenues, where there was space for a two-hundred-bed hospital.[18]

Planning for the new hospital focused on orthopaedics and did not deal with wider issues of child health and illness. It was thought, however, at the start of the hospital in 1922, that once neglected cases were dealt with, the need would be reduced. As has been demonstrated in many other health-care fields, this did not happen. Dr. M. Cody, Medical Superintendent, stated clearly that the aim of the hospital was "to take deformed and crippled children, and start them in life with a healthy body, and a healthy mind and an improved mentality."[19] Over 3,680 such patients had been cared for in the twenty-five years of the hospital's existence. Two major diseases at that time were tuberculosis and polio, both of which led to many deformities in children, and both figured significantly in the design of the new hospital. However, tuberculosis came under control soon after the discovery of streptomycin.[20] Epidemics of polio continued for a little longer, but eventually immunization led to the virtual disappearance of that disease.❖

References

1. *Annual Report*. Canadian Red Cross Society, Alberta Division, 1935, (note) p. 8-d.
2. *Annual Report*. Canadian Red Cross Society, Alberta Division, 1935.
3. Townsend, R.G., Lecture to Orthopaedic Surgeons. Calgary, October 1974, p. 2.
4. *Lent Report*, 1947, p. 112.
5. *The Calgary Herald*, April 29, 1939, p. 23.
6. Ibid.
7. Ken, via Dorothy Potts, personal communication.
8. *Lent Report*, 1947, p. 112.
9. *The Calgary Herald*, April 29, 1939, p. 23.
10. A. Hayes (*née* Ward), personal communication.
11. *The Calgary Herald*, January 26, 1957, p. 6.
12. *Annual Report*. Canadian Red Cross Society, Alberta Division, 1939, p. 5.
13. Dr. M. Cody's address, 1946.
14. *Lent Report*, 1947, p. 114.
15. Hardwick, E., E. Jameson and E. Tregillus. *The Science, the Art, and the Spirit: Medicine and Nursing in Calgary*. Century, Calgary, 1975, p. 139.

16. *Nursing Procedure Book*, p. 65.

17. *Annual Report*. Canadian Red Cross Society, Alberta Division, 1942, p. 5.

18. *The Calgary Herald*, September 11, 1945.

19. Address Dr. M. Cody, Revised, February 21, 1947, p. a.

20. After the serendipitous discovery of penicillin, there was a deliberate attempt to find other antibacterial agents. Waksman and associates examined soil actinomycetes (fungi) from 1939 onwards, and in 1943 identified the antibiotic streptomycin from a strain of Streptomyces griseus. This was highly effective in tuberculosis, although toxicity limited its use. Other effective antituberculosis drugs soon followed. (*Goodman & Gilman's The Pharmacological Basis of Therapeutics*. 9th ed., McGraw-Hill, New York, 1996)

Fond Memories

Margaret C. was born in 1927 in Redcliff, Alberta, premature (twenty-six weeks) and weighing less than two pounds. This was before there were any incubators, and she thinks that she was kept warm in front of the coal-burning fire. She had cerebral palsy due to prematurity, with spastic paralysis. Her father never accepted her, but Margaret was lucky to have a wonderful grandfather who encouraged her never to give up. He supported Margaret. For example, he made a wagon with a top on it, and trained the dog to pull her around town; he also made sure that she had speech therapy. In 1938, Margaret's mother took her to Dr. M. Cody at the Alberta Children's Hospital, but she was not admitted, as the hospital had never had a patient with such severe disabilities. However, her mother sat on the steps of the hospital for a week, and Margaret was finally admitted, although her mother had to sign a form allowing treatment at the choice of the physician, treatment that could be experimental. She felt that this was her daughter's only chance.

Her mother visited her in hospital once every six months, and whenever her mother came to the city to see Margaret, one of her brothers had to do all the housework and cooking. Margaret only found out about this many decades later when she asked her brother outright why he had never liked her. He then told her, and Margaret realized how hard it had been for him to be responsible for taking care of all of the needs of the family on these days.

When Margaret was first admitted to the hospital, she was placed in an isolation room which was actually the linen room and then a private room straight across from the operating room, the one room which scared all the children. Margaret was in this room by herself for almost six months. A canvas harness had been put on her but as she did not like it she cut it with scissors stolen from a nurse's uniform. Next the hospital staff tried a leather harness which took her longer to escape but she did manage. The third harness was made of steel, and even with her resourcefulness, she was unable to get out of that!

Margaret was not allowed to go to the hospital school but had goldfish to entertain her. She remembers the service club coming on Saturdays to take children who were well enough for a car ride and an ice cream. Each time they brought Margaret back another goldfish for her collection, and so her goldfish bowl filled up quickly. Listening to the radio was another treat, but this was only allowed for one hour a day, and only music at that.

After six months in the private room, Margaret was moved to the sun porch for another six months. Despite its name, the sun porch was really cold, and she was only brought into the house to be fed and to go to the bathroom. The cold was so intense that she hid under the feather quilt. Despite this, there was excitement on the sun porch because she could talk to the boys from the neighborhood.

Eventually braces were put on, and her hands were bandaged with red flannel bandages. This process was so painful that it remains in her memory. In those days, nothing was given for the pain, and she cried for about one week. After the first year in the hospital, she was allowed to go into the ward and also started exercises with the physiotherapist, Mildred Spreckley. She also encouraged girls to dress up in her room where she kept dress-up clothes. All the children loved her; their nickname for her was Speckle Bottoms.

Margaret was mischievous. All the girls would hide under her bed with the radio on at night and listen to hockey games and cowboy music. One night, she found a hole in the floor, which led to a complicated prank. She poured water down the hole just for the fun of it and did not know at that time where it ended up. One week later, she found out that it had landed exactly between the legs of a boy on the Boys' Ward, who kept telling the nurse that he was not wetting the bed and that the water was coming from the roof. The nurses did not believe him! The same sort of prank was recalled by Betty in 1981 during a reunion. She said, "if we wanted to get even with the boys on the floor below, we poured water along the (heating) pipes and it splashed on them in their beds."[1] Eventually Margaret was caught and was given the standard punishment of being put in the isolation room for one week and having to eat food that she did not like, a whole week's diet of turnips and porridge.

Margaret also worked out how to keep in touch with the boys. She hooked up a line from the Girls' Ward, and they pulled messages back and forth. In another game, the children regularly played ghosts running up and down the hallways with sheets over their heads.

Margaret remembers the wonderful moment when she got her first pair of shoes, and she used them immediately. She did not walk just on the flat floor surface but insisted on going down the steps of the hospital right away. It was no surprise that she fell; after regaining consciousness, she was sent to the isolation room for punishment, and no shoes, at least for a while.

One day outside on the porch, she discovered that the screen on the storage room was loose, and the window was open. Margaret always rose to a challenge, and as a nurses' conference was coming up, she organized all her friends on the conference day to take advantage of this wonderful opportunity. She went into the room and handed all the chocolate[2] to friends who were on the other side, and while this was going on Matron Reid came in to collect supplies. Margaret left as fast as possible. After this episode, the nurses wondered why the girls were not eating, and so they consulted the physicians who were in turn puzzled. All the girls were in relatively good health but were not hungry. This misdemeanor was also discovered, and she was in the isolation room again!

Margaret organized expeditions, even at night. For example, the children would go down the steps to the closest local store to buy candy and lipstick. Margaret remembers the brace shop in the basement which was called the "torment room" by the kids, who hated the room. For children who could not go down to the room, the brace maker would come up and do measurements at the bedside.

Margaret not only remembers all the tough times at the hospital, but also all the good times and realizes that these experiences made her the sort of person she is today.

When Margaret was interviewed recently, she said she still loves life and feels like sweet sixteen in her heart, although her old body did not feel that way anymore. She is now planning to move home for the 41st time.

References

1. *The Lethbridge Herald*, September 11, 1981, p. B4.
2. The authors have been unable to find the storage room where chocolate is kept in the present hospital, but believe an expedition led by children is more likely to be successful.

PART FOUR

THE THIRD HOSPITAL
1952–1972

❖❖❖❖❖❖❖❖❖❖❖❖❖

A Purpose-Built Hospital

T he entrance to the new building on Richmond Road was dramatic. There was a bas-relief figure on a pale concrete panel on both sides of the entrance. One of these figures was "Innocence" and the other "Little Boy Blue." Immediately beyond these panels and inside the main lobby were murals of animals and plants in white on a deep brownish rose background.[1] The enormous red cross had been moved from the previous building and was inlaid in the tile floor across from the library, where it remains to this day. The figures "Innocence" and "Little Boy Blue" are also still in the area of the Library. However, they are on the wall

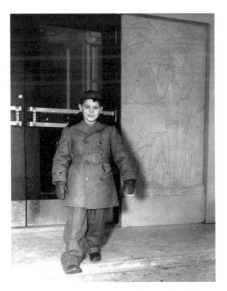

Entrance to new hospital.

away from the main hallway and almost obscured by temporary secretarial accommodation. The living quarters of the matron were across the hall of the main lobby.

This new building officially opened on March 3, 1951.[2] Patients moved in January 1952, but all this happened only after long hours had been spent planning, identifying a site and on the actual construction.

The first stage was to identify the site for the new building and, having done that, the Red Cross submitted an application to the City Land Department in September 1945 for allocation of the use of the land, which was approved the day it was submitted. Part of the chosen site was reserved

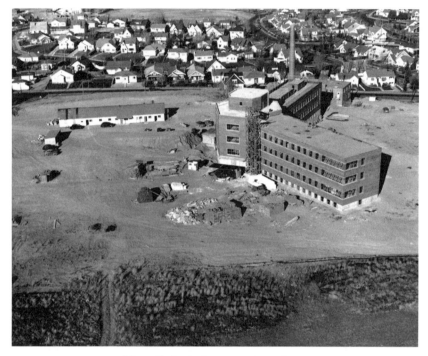

Hospital under construction.

for school purposes, but the Public School Board was prepared to release the land for a Crippled Children's Hospital. The site on which the hospital was to be built was a tax-free gift from the City of Calgary. On December 20, 1945, the deed was formally presented to the Alberta Division of the Red Cross.[3] Architects were selected at that time (W.S. Summerville of Toronto and J. Stevens of Calgary), and it was decided that the three-storey hospital was to be built of reinforced concrete with a warm-colored red brick facing. The first sod was turned on May 12, 1946, the anniversary of Florence Nightingale's birthday.

The cost estimate at the time of initial approval was $250,000 for a two-hundred-bed hospital, and the Red Cross had the necessary funds. However, by the time the deed was presented, only two months after the initial approval, the cost had risen to $300,000. Plans continued to evolve, and by November 1947, the intention was to have a 150-bed Junior Red Cross Children's Hospital eventually, but to build a 75- to 100-bed section immediately.[4] The reason for proceeding in phases was that costs had skyrocketed, and the available funds were no longer sufficient to build the whole building at once. The building fund at that time contained $765,000, but it was thought that another $500,000 would be needed for completion of the building.[5] Detailed plans were filed in 1948, and the city's Engineering Department approved a 100-bed, $820,000, new Red Cross Crippled Children's Hospital.[6] The plans were for a Y-shaped main building with wards and accommodation for many special departments, and also a small *L*-shaped building connected by an underground tunnel to the main building for staff, boiler house and laundry. By 1949, the number of beds and the costs had changed once more. This was now going to be a 119-bed hospital at a total cost of $1 million, which must have seemed a staggering amount.[7]

Great care was taken to make sure that this new hospital would be the most up-to-date on the continent. There were numerous special features in the design such as heated floors in the playroom, rounded baseboards in the corridors and a sundeck on the roof. This was a wide-open space with a brick wall designed to protect the hospital from the harsh Calgary winds, and a metal fence all around, which was later enclosed to become the solarium. Safety features in the plan included a fireproof building, with only the doors and cabinets to be made of wood. There were going to be three hundred windows, all wide and deep, double-glazed in aluminum frames, giving patients and staff a wide view of Calgary to the East and a panoramic view of the Rockies to the West. To quote the *Calgary Herald* in 1950, before the hospital was completed, "From the highest hilltop in Calgary, the new Junior Red Cross Crippled Children's Hospital looks down on a rapidly growing city, the rolling Foothills that form its boundaries and the snow capped Rocky Mountains to the West."[8] The cost escalated by the time of the official opening in 1951. The building cost was $1,133,000[9] and the plans for equipment were between $100,000 and $150,000. There were 119 beds in total, including twenty-five designated beds for polio patients in the South Wing on the third floor. As an extra, the nurses' stations came equipped with small refrigerators, so that cold drinks for patients could easily be obtained at night.

The Minister of Health, Dr. W.W. Cross, stated at the opening on March 3, 1951: "This is a great day for the many people who have contributed of time, money and effort ... for this kind of building."[10] The official name of the hospital at opening was the Alberta Red Cross Crippled Children's Hospital. "Alberta" had been added on March 2, 1951, to indicate that the hospital was meant to help children from areas outside Calgary, primarily southern Alberta, as well as those within the city. Mary Pinkham, who as a teenager had attended the opening of the first hospital in 1922 with her father Bishop Pinkham, was present. She was one of the original founders of the Junior Red Cross in Alberta and had remained very involved.

Much happened after the official opening: additional staff were trained; there was a wait for some equipment; other equipment was transferred;[11] and there was extensive planning for the operation of the new hospital.[12] The actual move took place in January 1952 in temperatures which never

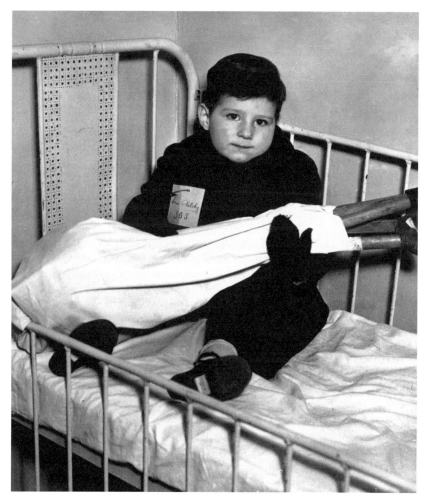

Ready for the move!

rose above −28° C! The move went smoothly, thanks to planning, volunteers and police assistance. Children were bundled into heavy clothing, and a name and number pinned to their clothes, corresponding to a number on their bed in the new hospital. The actual transport was in private cars by many volunteers who had helped throughout the years (such as the Kinsmen, the Active Club, the CHAS and other clubs) or by ambulance. Police officers made sure the roads were free for the cars to drive along a carefully planned route. The thirty-five walking patients were delivered in only thirteen minutes. Thirteen stretcher cases were brought later. Transporting the children within the hospital was made easier by the new elevator donated by the CHAS.

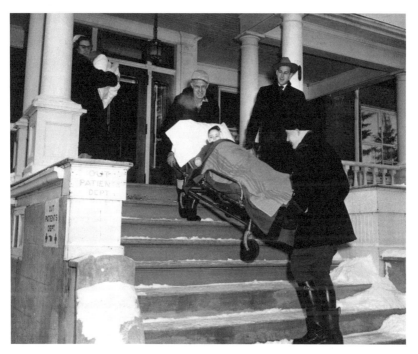

Out of the old hospital.

New patients, having been greeted in the warm entrance hall, went to an isolation room. There were two such rooms, and after a few days, the children moved on to the wards. The surgical suite was in the North Wing of the third floor, which is now office accommodation. Before the move, the only surgeries performed in the Children's Hospital were procedures such as tonsillectomies. Major surgery had been performed in other hospitals in the city, and this led to difficulties both for the children and the nurses. The children were uncomfortable being in another hospital and having to travel back and forth. The nurses were often so devoted that they visited "their children"[13] in these other city hospitals on their days off. Thus the ability to perform surgery and provide all post-operative care for the child in one and the same building was a major advantage. In 1952, 103 operations were performed. An anaesthetic room was available for both surgical suites, and this was designed to avoid the frightening experience of the child being taken directly to the operating room. As a spin-off benefit, this situation allowed more operations to be done in a day.

Once in the hospital, polio patients found themselves in brand new beds, called the Kenny bed. These beds were made in Eastern Canada. Once delivered to Calgary, they were re-designed along the lines of the beds used by Sister Kenny, and two carpenters here worked on the beds

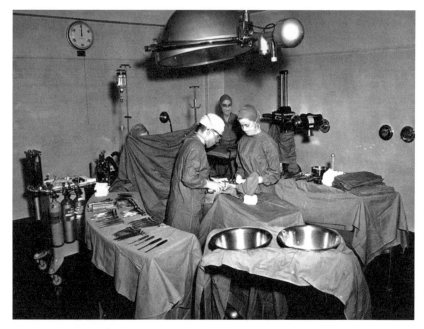

Operating theatre.

for over two weeks. They removed the metal parts, installed a flatboard instead of springs and added a trough at the end. Patients who were lying on their stomachs were thus able to lie flat with their feet protected in this trough.[14]

Important values of the old hospital were so much a part of the approach of the staff and volunteers that the same values automatically became part of life in the new hospital. These were clearly articulated by Clare Wallace in a radio broadcast in April 1946 called "Human Interest in an Orthopaedic Hospital."

> *First smiles, laughter and play – play organized and play impromptu, but always play. That is the normal atmosphere of childhood – the only atmosphere that can be conducive to child culture. To heal the child and ruin the personality – may God forbid – but it is almost humanly impossible to avoid just that in long illness, unless provision is made in a scientific up-to-date institution, especially staffed and especially equipped with all that goes to provide for not only average education, but the acceptance of handicap and the development of compensation.*[15]

That the hospital was successful in realizing this can be judged from Helen McArthur's remark that the hospital staff and administrators are to be praised for giving children "a hospital life that is as close as possible to a normal child life."[16] In the administrator's report on the new hospital, the children were reported to be "very happy indeed and it is a common sight everyday to see first one and then another ride tricycles and small automobiles, or push doll carriages up and down the long corridors."[17]

The children could not get away from school in this new building, just as they could not get away from education in the old building! There were three large classrooms, and provincial correspondence courses were followed. To attest to the dedication of the teachers and the students, no child had ever less than a *B* mark on a provincial test. Learning continued through occupational therapy. Some of the beautiful articles were sold, with the money going to the cost of the article and a portion of the remainder to the child. A regular accounting system was used, so that the child would learn the rudiments of saving and budgeting. Despite this, there was always time for fun, such as a picnic.

Out-patients had always been seen in the old hospitals, but the new hospital had an extended Out-patient Department. The East Wing was totally devoted to out-patients, and there was a clinic every Friday. In 1952, 878 patients were seen on 2,882 visits,[18] and each child was examined and, if required, braces were fitted. The parents were fully involved in the child's treatment and were given detailed instruction on home care. The administration of the Out-patient Clinic was handled totally by volunteers from the Junior League of Calgary, who played an important role in ensuring smooth running of the clinic. If an out-patient required tests, they were done in the laboratory on site.

There were many new features in the hospital. For example, there was a large formula room to prepare infant formula and a bottle-washing room. There was a dishwashing section for the older children and the staff. Food was prepared in the kitchen, and electrically heated wagons delivered it to the ward corridor still hot. On the top floor of this new building was a sewing room. There, groups of volunteers did the hospital sewing.[19] This was not mere repair work. They made much of the bed linen on site, a task which they had been doing for twenty years in the previous hospital. Medical records and the brace shop were in the basement of the building.

An outbreak of polio in the summer of 1952 led to the admission of one hundred patients. Margaret Baxter had to open the second floor for the first time to deal with the influx of patients.[20] There were too few staff to care for the children, and radio and newspapers helped in advertising for new staff. The following year, the outbreak of polio was so serious that it created a major emergency. In September, there were 160 patients,[21] 111 of whom had polio; the number of cases rose to an unprecedented high of 171. All available accommodation was used to such an extent that even the patient dining room was used as an eight-bed ward. Plans were also ready to turn the classrooms into wards should the epidemic

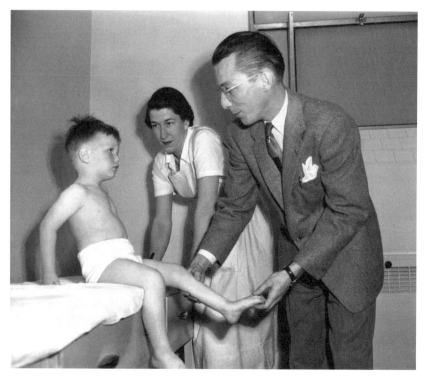

Dr. Sturdy examining a child in out-patients.

grow bigger. Throughout the whole of 1953, there were 323 in-patients, 213 of whom had polio. The average stay was 125.7 days, with 1,360 X-rays. In the same year, there were 3,708 out-patient visits by 1,147 patients.[22]

In the midst of all the turmoil, two movies were filmed. "They Dance Again" was sponsored by seven Alberta oilmen and the publicity department of the Canadian Red Cross and made by a Vancouver company. It stressed the home-like atmosphere of the hospital and the up-to-date facilities through the eyes of a polio patient who eventually gets to dance again. The other film "A Special Kind of Courage" was a fundraising film for the Easter Seal campaign funded by the CHAS and filmed in Calgary by Masters Studio. The film provided details such as the 4,000 pounds of wash each week and the 10,000 and more meals prepared every month for staff and patients. To compare these numbers to today, in 1996 the number of meals per month was roughly 15,000 for staff, and 7,500 for patients. Furthermore, the movie drew attention to the up-to-date techniques being used in the Operating Room and X-ray Department and the recent use of plastics in the fashioning of limbs, partly financed by the CHAS.

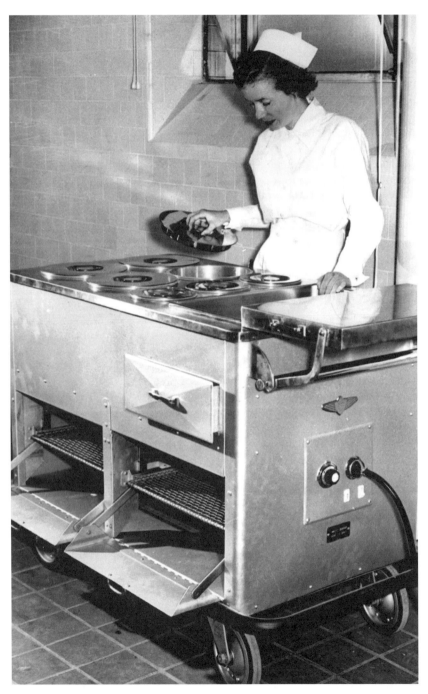

Food trolley.

There will never be a time when a hospital can be run without any worries about money, and even though the strong volunteer support continued, finances were still a concern, and the total operating cost for the hospital in 1952 was $276,461.37. Nevertheless, in this financially lean period, the Red Cross was so impressed by the staff that they increased nurses salaries by $15[23] which meant that the gross total salary per month for a registered nurse was $190.

The hospital was well designed, but changes and additions were needed to keep abreast of developments in paediatric care. For example, there was an addition to the building in 1955, with the construction of the solarium and auditorium on the former play deck. The CHAS donated the receipts from their annual Easter Seal campaign to this extension, which was opened officially in 1956. In October 1955, the Alberta Red Cross Children's Hospital was given full accreditation by the Joint Commission of Accreditation of Hospitals for the United States and Canada. This honor is attained by hospitals that provide the best in medical, nursing and hospital services.[24]

To honor all the dedicated men and women who had contributed to the Children's Hospital, a plaque was unveiled in 1955 that recognized those who had devoted time and skill to the crippled youngsters. This can still be seen in the hospital.

References

1. "Calgary's Modern Red Cross Hospital," *The Canadian Hospital*, August 1951, pp. 29-31.
2. Booklet for the opening of the third hospital. Alberta Junior Red Cross Crippled Children's Hospital.
3. *The Calgary Herald*, December 20, 1945.
4. *Minutes*. Executive Committee, Alberta Division, Canadian Red Cross Society, November 21, 1947, p. 9.
5. *Annual Report*. Canadian Red Cross Society, Alberta Division, 1947.
6. *The Calgary Herald*, June 23, 1948.
7. *The Calgary Herald*, July 8, 1949.
8. *The Calgary Herald*, December 2, 1950.
9. *The Calgary Herald*, February 12, 1951.
10. *The Calgary Herald*, March 5, 1951.
11. *The Calgary Herald*, January 15, 1952.
12. *The Calgary Herald*, January 16, 1952.
13. Booklet for the opening of the third hospital. Alberta Red Cross Crippled Children's Hospital.
14. *The Calgary Herald*, August 28, 1951.
15. "Human Interest in an Orthopaedic Hospital." Transcript prepared for Clare Wallace's radio broadcast, April 1946.
16. Helen McArthur, National Director, Nursing Services, Canadian Red Cross and President, Canadian Nurses Association, in *The Calgary Herald*, December 13, 1952.
17. Long, R.J. "Administrator's Report." *In Annual Report*. Canadian Red Cross Society, Alberta Division, 1951, p. 44.
18. *Annual Report*. Canadian Red Cross Society, Alberta Division, 1952, p. 20.

19. *Annual Report*. Canadian Red Cross Society, Alberta Division, 1950, p. 53.
20. *The Volunteer*, 3(7) (September 1952): 1, 3.
21. *The Calgary Herald*, September 23, 1953.
22. *Annual Report*. Canadian Red Cross Society, Alberta Division, 1953, pp. 5, 39.
23. Personnel Committee Meeting, July 10, 1952.
24. *Annual Report*. Canadian Red Cross Society, Alberta Division, 1955, p. 27.

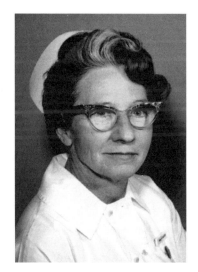

Margaret Baxter

returned to Calgary as Assistant Director of Nursing at the Alberta Red Cross Crippled Children's Hospital and succeeded Florence Reid as Director of Nursing in 1952.

She was responsible for many innovations such as the affiliation program for student nurses in orthopaedic training and an educational program for staff nurses given by physicians and surgeons on staff.

In 1956, the Red Cross asked her to join a team of six nurses from Canada to go to Europe to assist in the camps caring for Hungarian refugees.

She worked at the Alberta Children's Hospital until 1965, when she went to the Rockyview Hospital, where she remained as Director of Nursing until her retirement.

Margaret Baxter graduated from the University of Alberta Hospital in Edmonton and was on staff there until she joined the RCAF in 1942 as a nursing sister. She was discharged in 1946, went to Edmonton to work with Dr. F.H.H. Mewburn, then went to Boston University for further training. She worked for a short time in Alberta, then became Supervisor of the Junior Red Cross Wing at the Regina General Hospital. She

Alberta Children's Hospital Society

Through the 1950s, discussion of the role of government in health care and to what extent the system should be publicly financed continued throughout Canada. The Government of Alberta, like that of other provinces, had already decided to pay a large part of hospitalization through taxation. The Alberta Division of the Red Cross kept a close watch on its finances and realized that it was spending $200,000 a year more in Alberta than it was receiving. The difference was expected to increase, as the hospital was becoming busier. Also the Red Cross was developing a new role and vision for itself, and the provision of a service for the collection and distribution of blood was beginning to dominate its activities. The budget reflected the increasing cost of this service. Moreover, the Red Cross was anxious to maintain a traditional role, helping out immediately in disasters. The low level of reserve funds meant that a prompt response to a major crisis would not be possible.

Thus, by 1957, the hospital was financed by grants from the province, direct donations from the public, donations via other organizations and the Red Cross annual campaign. The *Poliomyelitis Sufferers' Act* allowed the province to increase its grants to $10.25 per day for polio cases and $3.40 per day for others. Costs were increasing at a greater pace than reimbursement; in 1957, the cost per patient per day was $12.24, and the cost per patient would soon be fourteen dollars per day to operate. The proposed grant from the province was ten dollars per patient per day. Families of the patients would pay $1.80, and the rest needed to be covered by donations.[1]

With the shift in the focus of the Red Cross, it made sense to turn over the management of the hospital, and the property itself, to a new society, the Alberta Crippled Children's Hospital Society, which was formed on January 1, 1958, and had a Board with both Red Cross members and other interested individuals.[2] This was a non-profit organization, dedicated to the management of the hospital and the care of children. There was an agreement to continue to care for orthopaedically handicapped children; the Alberta Crippled Children's Hospital[3] was to be continued as long as the need was apparent, and indeed expansion beyond orthopaedic services could be considered.[4]

This was the beginning of a special era for the Alberta Children's Hospital when there was a greater degree of autonomy than at any other time in the hospital's existence. The previous management committee, although devoted to the Alberta Children's Hospital, was still a subdivision of the Red Cross and, after 1972, the successor to the Alberta Children's Hospital Society was the Alberta Children's Hospital Board, appointed by, and responsible to, the provincial government.

The Directors of the Red Cross, with Mervyn G. Graves as Chairman, turned over a hospital which was operating 124 of its 156 beds. The new

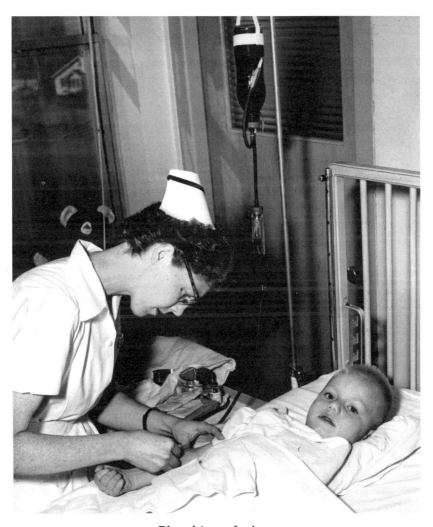

Blood transfusion.

society, at its first meeting on December 18, 1957, elected Mervyn Graves as President. The first few meetings dealt not only with everyday issues but with the "underuse" of the hospital. The large polio epidemics were over and there were still children with polio-induced deformities who required care, but all of the orthopaedic cases taken together were insufficient to use the hospital's facilities to their maximum. Other surgeons (general; eye, ear, nose and throat; and plastic) admitted children for surgery and post-operative care. Despite this, the number of empty beds led to consideration of many different solutions, including admitting general paediatric (non-surgical) patients. Thus there were discussions with

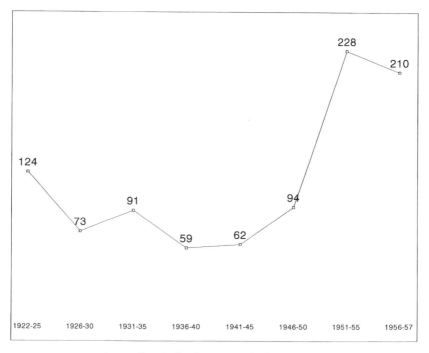

In-patient discharges, 1922–1957.

the other hospitals that admitted children and with the paediatricians. By the end of 1958, six paediatricians were on staff,[5] but they admitted few children because of concerns about the care of acutely ill children in a hospital without physicians on the premises twenty-four hours a day. Discussions with the Calgary General Hospital and the Holy Cross Hospital about the relocation of some interns to the Alberta Children's Hospital were unsuccessful. The medical staff pressed for more operating-room equipment, increased laboratory and pathology services, and better X-ray services, all of which were necessary if the hospital was to admit children with acute illnesses.

The new policy of "open admissions" came into effect on January 1, 1959. However, the door was not yet fully open. There were restrictions: patients were to be sixteen years of age or less; no acute infectious cases were to be admitted; no psychiatric cases requiring restraint were allowed. Some of these policies were developed by the new administrator, S.V. Pryce, appointed on June 24, 1958, to replace O.H. Clusiau. In a reaction to these new policies, the mayor stated that this would "relieve pressure on the General Hospital which has a waiting list."[6]

There were new arrangements for payment. The federal *Hospital Insurance and Diagnostic Services Act* (1957) authorized payment for hospitals, laboratory tests and X-rays. The cost of hospital care was

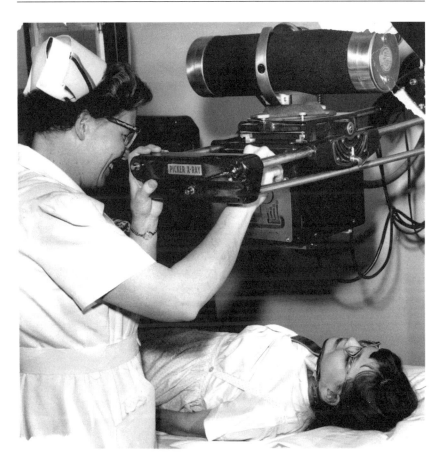

Lying still for an X-ray.

shared between the federal and provincial governments and funds transferred to the Alberta Crippled Children's Hospital. As in the provincial municipal hospitals, a small sum was charged to all patients and collected from those who were able to pay. From now on, all Alberta children were eligible for admission, but bills were sent routinely to parents. The hospital would not confine itself to in-patient care and would continue its many special services. Some of these special services would require specific fundraising, but it was not thought that the sums requested would be large. Indeed, by late 1959, it was expected that fundraising organizations such as the CHAS would no longer be required, inaccurate as this subsequently proved to be.

The word "crippled" was part of the hospital name, and, when first used in 1949, was still an acceptable way of describing children and adults with disabilities. Only a few years later, many parents of such children disliked the negative connotation of the word, were uncomfortable

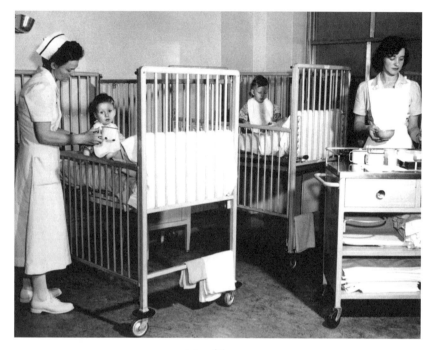

Mealtime.

with its use in general and wanted the word removed from the official name of the hospital. Not everyone agreed that the word was the problem. For example, Matron Florence Reid felt that the real issue was an acceptance of limitations on the child's future and that a disability, properly handled, could be the foundation for the child's success or, as the proverb says, "The sickness of the body may prove the health of the soul." These positive concepts were behind the phrase "physically challenged," which came into use decades later. The paediatricians supported the parents and requested the Board to rename the hospital. The Board agreed and resolved to remove the word "crippled" from the title in February 1959, formally agreed to use the title "Alberta Children's Hospital" in September 1959, and all legal steps were completed by November 17, 1959, when the hospital first had its present name.[7]

The hospital continued to concentrate on the philosophy of focussing on the whole child. The desire to do more than improve the disability remained, with a routine and programs designed to make up for what was missed by not being at home. Every effort was made to see the child had a normal, full and satisfying life. There was hardly any change in the regular routine of care.[8] The children were awake at 7 a.m. with breakfast at 7:15 a.m., and bathed and dressed immediately afterwards. Great care was taken to give the children clothes of different styles which they could

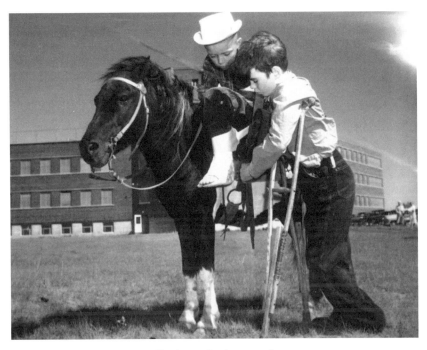

"Let me help you."

pick out for themselves. This was a further effort to achieve as normal a life as possible. The children were expected to attend school in the morning and afternoon with the appropriate breaks. Wherever possible, patients went to one of the school rooms, but patients confined to bed were visited by a teacher. Some patients would still be in the hospital for many years, doing their entire schooling there from grade one to grade twelve. The meals were served in the dining room from colorful dishes. The nurses paid attention to nutrition and watched carefully to see that the children ate their meals properly, but treats were also allowed. Gum, for example, was allowed every so often with a lesson on etiquette as to how to get rid of it! The children were also given vitamins. Every morning, the nurses would come and hand them out, patiently waiting until they were swallowed. However, once the nurse moved on to the next bed, children might spit them out and put them in the hollow legs of their beds. Much later, when intravenous poles did not fit anymore, the nurses found that the legs were filled with vitamins! The children may not have had many trips but, for example, instead of going on a trail ride, horses would be brought to the hospital.

Visiting hours were extremely limited, one hour every Wednesday and Sunday, and only direct relatives over the age of sixteen were admitted. There were never more than two visitors at one time. Even these hours could be limited further by the staff. "In rare cases where a visit upsets a child, visits are halted until the little patient gets used to the idea of seeing Mommy and Daddy infrequently."[9] The hardships and difficulties were recognized by creating the position of Director of Special Services (forerunner of Social Work), responsible for maintaining contact with out-of-town patients. It would have been more satisfactory for parents to spend time with their children and see how they were progressing. By this time, the seminal work by John Bowlby on the importance of parent, especially maternal, and child attachment and the dangers of separating children from their parents was becoming widely recognized.[10] Numerous studies and articles on the harmful effects of hospital visiting policies were leading many institutions to liberalize their visiting hours. In Canada, Montreal Children's Hospital was a leader in this area, but the Hospital for Sick Children in Toronto lagged behind. There, it was as late as 1961 before daily visiting (three hours in the afternoon) was introduced, and 1965 before there was all-day visiting (11 a.m. to 8 p.m.).[11]

In Calgary, the various parent and professional groups had many different attitudes towards visiting. For example, some nurses pushed for more extensive visiting, while others felt that the parents might interfere with the high level of care a professional could offer a child. Some physicians were concerned that parents might bring infection into the hospital, whereas others were aware of the importance of maintaining parent-child bonds. The paediatricians brought this issue before the Board, supported by senior nurses, and daily visiting was finally approved in 1965.[12]

For preschool children, daily visiting was 10 a.m. to 12 noon and 2 p.m. to 6 p.m., and for school-age children was 4 p.m. to 8 p.m., Monday to Saturday, and 10 a.m. to 8 p.m., Sundays and holidays. Sometimes restrictions were imposed by the hospital staff,[13] and it was probably a long time before there was full acceptance and implementation of the new rules. Now visiting throughout the twenty-four hours is not only allowed, it is strongly encouraged. There is still debate, but now the issues are whether or not extended family members can visit on the same basis as parents.

In the Alberta Children's Hospital, between 1958 and 1959, there was a marked change in workload (see table).

	Admissions	Discharges	Registered Out-patients	Minor Surgery
1958	274	268	758	46
1959	1344	1306	794	844

This was largely due to a deliberate attempt to increase the number of patients by encouraging physicians to bring their patients to the Alberta Children's Hospital. The success of the policy is shown by the enormous change in minor surgery, of which 752 cases (89.09%) were tonsillecto-mies. This continued for many years and led to accusations that the hos-pital was "for tonsils," which to some extent lowered its reputation in medical circles. Children who had minor surgery stayed in the hospital for such a short time that the bed occupancy was still only 65.9 percent in 1959, despite the large increase in cases. There was little change in the number of out-patients at first, and the large increase in the number of clinics and major focus on ambulatory care would come later.

In 1958, during internal discussions to widen the scope of the Alberta Children's Hospital, there were many other medical developments in Calgary and the rest of the province. The Health Minister, J.D. Ross, and his staff were reviewing sites for a new provincial hospital in Calgary (the future Foothills Hospital). The site occupied by the Alberta Children's Hospital was one of the suggestions, and the Minister felt that if this site was used, the present unit could be used as a children's wing. The actual choice of the future Foothills Hospital site was said to be made when J.D. Ross visited the administrator's office in the Alberta Children's Hos-pital to discuss expansion of that hospital. During this discussion, he looked out the window and said "What you need is another general hos-pital. That open land on the hill over there would be a good place for it."[14] Dr. Ross's view was that the new hospital would have a minimum number of paediatric beds, which the Alberta Children's Hospital Board wanted to be for short-term care only. The Foothills Hospital was eventu-ally opened in 1966, and its agreed facilities for general paediatric cases led to much discussion and controversy through the 1970s and into the early 1980s.

Discussion of the expansion of the Alberta Children's Hospital, which started in 1958, led to a formal brief on May 28, 1964. One month later, the Minister of Health approved in principle an increase in total capacity to three hundred beds, at a cost of $2 million. The provincial government also wanted units for the multihandicapped in Calgary and Edmonton and were prepared to place one hundred of these beds at the Foothills Hospital site. The Calgary Paediatric Society was not satisfied with the suggestions and wanted most of the paediatric beds to be on one site. This group felt that paediatric units in general hospitals were "satellites of adults facilities ... not totally oriented towards the care of children."[15] However, it pointed out that an increase in beds alone at the Alberta Children's Hospital site would lead to major problems, as support serv-ices were already insufficient. Thus the demand for more operating rooms, greater laboratory capacity and a larger X-ray department became more insistent.

The issues of expansion were complex, and the Board called a special meeting in March 1965 to discuss this topic. As a result, the administra-tor (S.V. Pryce), two architects and two Board members visited several

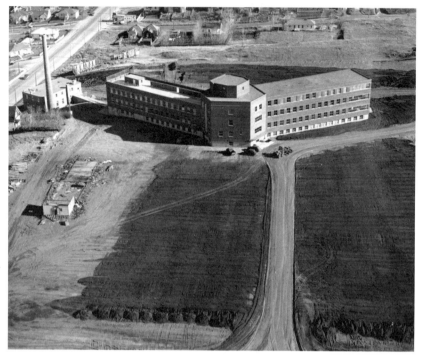

Work on the site.

children's hospitals in Canada and the U.S.A. to gather more information. Principles developed were: any children's hospital should jealously guard and maintain its autonomy; the hospital should develop from a community hospital to a specialized children's unit; and when the new Medical School in Calgary opened, the Alberta Children's Hospital should be the paediatric teaching unit. It was also resolved that there should be research facilities, and a long-range plan should include the development of a child health centre on or adjacent to the present site.[16]

During the early part of 1966, great progress was made. Detailed plans were approved by the government, and staff were recruited to help in planning. Attempts to acquire the house on the northwest corner, which had started in 1964, continued. Part of the site was cleared and used as fill in the construction of a new highway nearby (now Crowchild Trail). The Alberta Children's Hospital Board also met with the University of Alberta in Calgary. By the end of that year, Dr. W.A. Cochrane had been appointed Dean of the Faculty of Medicine of The University of Calgary, and the Board was anxious to meet with him to discuss the site of the hospital and the details of the plans. The end result was that the architects were placed "on hold" while the whole concept of development was revisited.

The news in 1968 was not good. Early in the year, the Minister of Health stopped all new hospital construction in the province. Later in the year, plans of the medical school for paediatrics at Foothills Hospital were revealed at a meeting attended by the Alberta Children's Hospital Board and architect, the administrator of Foothills Hospital (L.R. Adshead), Dr. Cochrane and the Deputy Minister. At the time of the discussion, the medical school occupied two floors at the Foothills Hospital. When permanent accommodation for the medical school was complete, these floors would become available for patient care and would allow an additional one hundred paediatric beds, to give a total of 170 beds. This would enable Foothills Hospital to be a major paediatric referral centre. Dr. Cochrane suggested the Alberta Children's Hospital should continue as an orthopaedic and rehabilitation facility and develop an assessment and educational centre. There was general concern in paediatric circles at this fragmentation of services and proliferation of expensive paediatric facilities in each hospital.[17]

The concept of a child health centre was still strongly supported by the Alberta Children's Hospital Board which felt the best site was at Foothills Hospital. When Dr. Ross said this was not possible, the present Alberta Children's Hospital site was accepted. The preservation of a role for the Alberta Children's Hospital in active treatment was important, and there was willingness to accept the multihandicapped program, provided it did not prejudice existing programs. Dr. G. Holman had been appointed Head of Paediatrics at The University of Calgary and also appointed a consultant by the provincial government. He presented his suggestions to the Alberta Children's Hospital Board, which included a child health centre based on ambulatory care with as many beds as would be required to support good care. The Child Health Centre should have its "own autonomous board" made up of individuals from the existing Alberta Children's Hospital Board, The University of Calgary and consumers (parents). If autonomy was not possible at the Foothills site, the Child Health Centre should be elsewhere. The units at Calgary General, Holy Cross and Rockyview hospitals should not grow but be linked with a network centered at the Child Health Centre. He also suggested that the agencies dealing with children co-operate under the leadership of the Alberta Children's Hospital. It was important that the province fund a study of total paediatric and adolescent needs along with a financial evaluation.

Financial considerations stalled the planning process, and throughout 1970 and 1971, the government gave warnings of the financial problems it faced. Nevertheless, the government was still interested in developing programs for the multihandicapped, which would include the relocation of the Cerebral Palsy Clinic from SAIT. The Alberta Children's Hospital Board was also interested in a Diagnostic, Assessment and Treatment Centre and discussion on this specific development started in 1971,

George Lancaster
and Mervyn Graves

These two gentlemen served on the boards of the Red Cross, the Alberta Children's Hospital Society and the Alberta Children's Hospital Foundation and gave unsparingly of their time. George Lancaster served the various boards for fifty-three years and Mervyn Graves for fifty-seven years, and both participated in many important decisions.

George Lancaster, a well-known businessman in Calgary, was present at the opening of the hospital in 1922. He originally came to the Alberta Children's Hospital from the Red Cross, when he started to become involved in the Red Cross Military Convalescent Hospital, after World War I. His love was with the Alberta Children's Hospital from its origin in 1922. He was Chairman of the Property Committee in the second hospital, when extra fire slides had to be installed. One of his other functions was Chair of the Bequest Committee, and he remarked that bequests often came in up to twenty-five years after children had been here. He served consecutively on many boards until 1975, when he was on the Board of Directors of the Alberta Children's Hospital Foundation.

Merv Graves also gave unprecedented service to the Alberta Children's Hospital for more than fifty years. He was born, raised and educated in Calgary and obtained his Chartered Accountancy degree in 1931. He achieved prominence in his profession and was president of the Institute of Chartered Accountants of Alberta (1941) and president of the Canadian Institute of Chartered Accountants (1968-69). Merv had many volunteer involvements and again achieved distinction as president and governor of the Kinsmen's Club of Calgary (1939-40), potentate of the Al Azhar Shrine Temple (1962) and director of the Francis F. Reeve Foundation (1965-83). His long connection with ACH started in 1930 when he joined the Kinsmen's Club and became interested in their service work at the Red Cross Crippled Children's Hospital. He was chairman of the Red Cross Crippled Children's Hospital (1951-59) while it was operated by the Red Cross. He then became the president of the new Alberta Children's Hospital Society (1959) and continued until the government took over the hospital in 1972. Thus he oversaw two major transitions in the life of ACH and initiated the planning process that led to the Child Health Centre. Often the meetings he chaired (as a volunteer) were in the evening and continued until midnight. He was seen as a quiet

❖❖❖❖❖❖❖❖❖❖❖❖❖

but effective leader. As a member of the Kinsmen's Club, he attended almost every Christmas Party for children. When he was unable to attend because of illness on one occasion, it was noted that up to that point he had been to thirty-seven consecutive parties.

Merv Graves was the first president of the Alberta Children's Hospital Foundation (1972-82), became chairman in 1982-83 and remained on the ACHF Board until the year of his death (1987).

His long and devoted service is recognized in the newly established Merv Graves Educational Fellowship awarded by the Alberta Children's Hospital Foundation.

although the report would not be available until the Alberta Children's Hospital had again undergone a change of owners (the new owners being the government).

These discussions were held against a background of increasing knowledge of the many diseases that affect children. The infant mortality rate continued to fall, and in 1959 was 28.4 per 1,000 live births, two thirds of these deaths occurring in the first four weeks of life. There were even more dramatic reductions in the death rate of children beyond the age of four weeks. There had been a dramatic drop in the number of deaths due to tuberculosis with the advent of effective chemotherapy.[18] Deaths from other infectious diseases had also fallen dramatically. These trends, the falling death rates and the drop in the frequency of infectious diseases, were to lead to a recognition in the next decade that there were many other problems in childhood that required attention, principally chronically handicapping conditions. Ironically, these had formed the bulk of the workload of the Alberta Children's Hospital, particularly if surgery was required. There were many chronic handicapping conditions not amenable to rapid or full recovery, and as paediatricians developed an interest in these conditions, the phrase "new paediatrics" was coined.

The response to concern about chronic disease was slow but definite. The long-standing Orthopaedic Clinic was joined by Cleft Palate, Dental and Orthoptic clinics (1960), Pre-school Deaf (1963) and Juvenile Amputee (1965) clinics. There were other clinics: the SAIT Cerebral Palsy clinic already mentioned and another for Cystic Fibrosis at the Calgary General Hospital.

Children not only continued to receive excellent care at the Alberta Children's Hospital but also had new treats. A Coca-Cola machine was purchased in 1962 for $432, but this was not benevolence alone. It was expected to generate revenue of $47 per month. The many volunteers worked hard to make life pleasant and even took a group to the Ice Capades one year. The Kinsmen still had a Christmas party every year, and the thirty-eighth annual party on December 1967 was noteworthy as the first one Mervyn Graves had missed! These entertainments were not enough for some of the teenagers who got into mischief. After a hospital inspection, the Department of Public Health expressed concern about patients who were "teenagers ... who do smoke."[19]

During the 1950s and 1960s, there were groups of barbers who cut the children's hair every week for free. They needed written permission from their parents though, because some children would try anything not to have their hair cut. Dental care was also provided.

Most of the day-to-day care was provided by the nurses. This not only included care for the children, but also for the twenty-two birds and many goldfish around the hospital. Since the children were allowed to keep pets, many had birds in cages. The cleaning of the cages and feeding of the birds was the responsibility of the nurses. Woe to the nurse who let a bird escape and great fun for everyone chasing it through the ward's two corridors.

There was considerable turnover of nurses, not due to bird-care. A detailed study in 1962 shows thirty changes out of a staff of forty-two graduate nurses and sixteen changes out of the thirty-two other nurses. The main reasons were pregnancy, moving away, marriage and taking a new position. Nurses came from other hospitals for training in paediatric orthopaedic nursing, and although the Calgary General Hospital terminated its agreement in 1960, close contact remained with the Holy Cross Hospital, St. Michael and Municipal Hospitals in Lethbridge and the Medicine Hat Hospital. In 1966, a new era in nurse education began when Mount Royal College started to train nurses and sought affiliation with the Alberta Children's Hospital.

Relations between the Board and the nurses were not always smooth, and the Board had several rounds of negotiations with the Graduate Nurses Association and the Alberta Association of Registered Nurses (AARN). Eventually the Board participated in province-wide negotiations. Pay raises were granted, but even at the top level of the profession, nurses were not high on the pay scale in the hospital. For example, the prosthetist was paid more than the Director of Nursing.

During the period 1958-71, many long-standing employees left. Florence Reid retired in 1961, and the Board granted a pension, but made it clear that there was no obligation to do so and indeed reduced the payment in 1965 when she started to receive a pension from the federal government. Margaret Baxter succeeded Florence Reid, and she left in 1965 and was succeeded by Dorothy Potts. The pharmacist, Betty Laycraft retired in 1966, but returned as Director of Pharmacy in 1971 before retiring again in 1978. The school lost two long-service employees in 1967, M.M. Gillespie, the principal, retired after nineteen years of service, and Frances McClure retired from teaching after twenty-eight years. There were losses due to death, including Mrs. Andrews, the Medical Records Librarian, who was planning for a medical library at the time of her death. The most notable retirements of the 1960s were the Mathers, father and son. When James Mather, Sr., was seventy-seven, the Board felt that "one of his boys" should take over, but the delicate matter of persuading him to retire dragged on. He retired in 1960 at age seventy-nine and was granted a small pension. He died at the age of eighty-seven in 1968. Jack took over, but running the service was not his forte, and he returned to the construction of braces and prostheses in 1963. He continued for a short time but left the hospital in 1965 after twenty-seven years service and now lives in retirement in Edmonton.

New staff came, and many of the medical staff gave long service to the hospital (some are still active). The small band of paediatricians were joined by M. Pearson in 1960, and later A.J. Kavanagh, M.D. Heimbach, D.H.R. Truscott, G.M. Watkins, R.J. Sommerville and R.M. Vaswani. Two orthopaedic surgeons who gave notable service were Glen Edwards and W.M. Hunter. Glen Edwards came in 1960 and played an important role in setting up an orthopaedic training program.[20] J.M. Hunter saw the hospital being built as a schoolboy, came on staff in 1966 and still contributes to orthopaedic services. Children had much more contact with the orthopaedic residents, whom they saw several times per day, than with the staff surgeons, and often close relationships sprang up between the children and the trainee orthopaedic surgeons.

Some of the changes indicated that the organization was becoming more impersonal. Traditionally, the Alberta Children's Hospital supplied free coffee at breaks. As the other Calgary hospitals charged the staff for coffee, the Alberta Children's Hospital followed suit in 1968 to save an estimated $3,000 per year.

Most of the treatment was low key, and the surgery was uneventful and successful. There were exceptions. In 1963, there was a near-fatality when a girl having routine orthopaedic surgery had a cardiac arrest. Her chest was quickly opened, and following cardiac massage, she recovered. The expenses, including special nurses for five days, were heavy for a family that was not well off, and the Board waived some of the charges.

There were other fundamental changes in health care that affected everyone, but their impact was to take many years to fully understand and still provokes controversy. The most radical of these were two federal acts regarding medical care. The first was the *Hospital Insurance and Diagnostic Services Act* (1957), followed by the *Medical Care Act* (1966), which led to physician payment. These were, strictly speaking, provincial issues, but the federal government transferred money each year to match provincial spending on hospitals and physicians.

This system, dominated by hospital care as the main service to be provided and physicians as the main decision makers and gatekeepers, has so influenced the thinking of the Canadian public and politicians, that reform to include other professions in decision-making or to provide care outside the hospital has been difficult.❖

References

1. Annual Report. Canadian Red Cross Society, Alberta Division, 1957, p. 13.
2. Ibid., p. 35.
3. *The Volunteer*, 8(2) (December 1957): 1.
4. *The Calgary Herald*, December 3, 1957.
5. Paediatricians were J.D. Birrell, A.C. Cody, R.C.B. Corbett, J.U. Crichton, G.O. Prieur, H.W. Price.
6. *The Calgary Herald*, December 3, 1957.
7. *Minutes*. Alberta Children's Hospital Board, February 24, 1959; September 15, 1959; November 17, 1959.
8. Alberta Red Cross Hospital, Child-care booklet for parents, 1957.
9. Ibid.
10. Bowlby, John. *Maternal Care and Mental Health*. World Health Organization, 1951. In John Bowlby, *Child Care and the Growth of Love*. Penguin, London, 1953.
11. Young, Judith. "Changing attitudes towards families of hospitalized children from 1935 to 1975: A case study." *Journal of Advanced Nursing*, 17 (1992): 1422-1429.
12. *Minutes*. Alberta Children's Hospital Board, March 25, 1965.
13. D.K. Stephure, personal communication.
14. Address by Dr. T.A. Richardson, October 1987.
15. Calgary Paediatric Society, Brief presented to the Alberta Children's Hospital Board, October 29, 1964.
16. Alberta Children's Hospital Board, October 18, 1965.
17. *Minutes*. Alberta Children's Hospital Board, September 26, 1968.
18. The word "chemotherapy" was originally used for antibiotics. It is almost never used in that sense now, but to denote anti-cancer drugs.
19. Letter from the Department of Public Health to the Hospital Inspector, April 1, 1970.
20. Edwards, Glen E., and D.B. Harkness. *Life Near the Bone*, Ronald's Printing, Calgary, 1991.

Background information

Canadian Encyclopedia, 2nd ed., Hurtig, Edmonton, s.v. "health care."

Life in the new hospital

During the polio outbreak of 1952 and 1953, the hospital was at the peak of its activities, and, after the outbreak, the hospital was quiet, and thus memories vary.

Although they appreciated that the hospital was built with children in mind, patients who moved to the new hospital in 1952 nevertheless felt the complete loss of the home-like atmosphere of the second hospital. Those who were admitted for the first time in 1952, however, had no direct knowledge of the previous hospitals and appreciated the love and warmth of this hospital.

Dale was one of those admitted in 1952, and her most vivid memory is that all the children were dressed in red, though what she is really remembering is not red clothing but the result of treatment. All were wrapped in hot packs as part of the Sister Kenney treatment, and then covered with square pieces of red

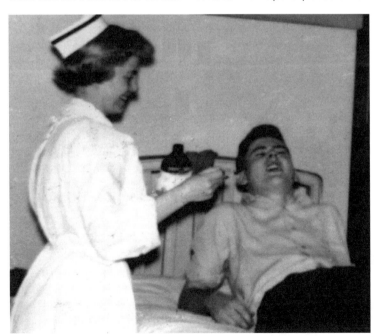

Cod liver oil.

cloth. She shares most of the following memories with Reny.

The hospital routine was strict. Every morning, as soon as the children woke up, they would get dressed, either in clothes provided by the hospital or, if supplied by their parents, the clothes had to be taken home for washing. The children were given a teaspoon of cod liver oil in the morning immediately before they went to the schoolrooms. After morning lessons, they all had lunch. The same hot meals were always served on the same days of the week, for example, Friday was always fish day.

Visiting days when Dale was in the hospital were Wednesday and Friday, but only for parents. She always wanted to see her siblings and her friends, and she had to go up to the sundeck, lean over and shout down to the street. There was lots of noise as children were shouting to and from the sundeck. As Dale improved and felt better, her parents got permission to take her for a ride. However, she could not be taken home even for a couple of minutes, and her parents had to make a strict promise to that effect.

She could only be driven around the neighborhood.

The staff were friendly, and the matron, Margaret Baxter, knew all the children by name and always had time to talk to Dale, Reny and the other children. There was something special for each day to relieve what could otherwise have been a monotonous existence. The most important day for Dale was movie day, held in the large physiotherapy room, when most of the children lay on the floor to watch their favorite movies, western movies provided by the Kinsmen.

Bill was admitted in 1962 to a hospital which was much less busy as the polio epidemics had passed. Many children were still admitted for orthopaedic treatment for deformities resulting from their polio or cerebral palsy. Bill had cerebral palsy, and his first admission was for one month to try and lengthen the cords in his right leg. This was only partially successful, and in 1968, he was admitted for two months when a further attempt was made to lengthen the cords to the heel and to the hip in his right leg. The operation helped quite a bit and allowed him to move around, although he still walks on the toes of his right foot.

Bill came from Hanna, Alberta, and his parents were not able to visit often but always managed to be there when he came out of surgery. In three months, he saw his brother through a window only twice. Despite this, he has great memories as there were always things to do and people to offer entertainment, such as a magician and clowns. Bill also remembers helping the nurse and the surgeon. Now, as a parent of a child with a chronic illness, Bill attends the DAT Centre and the Emergency Department and finds the ACH "one of the best hospitals in the world" with good care in Emergency or clinic. David was admitted in 1969, at a time when the hospital certainly was not busy. He was in grade ten, he had had hip pain, had seen a number of physicians in Lethbridge and had been given physiotherapy. None of the treatments had been helpful and a chiropractor was consulted. The family physician ordered more X-rays, which showed slipped femoral epiphyses. David was referred to Dr. Townsend who was acknowledged as by far the best orthopaedic surgeon in the Prairies. In the hospital, he had no involvement in his own care. None of the physicians would discuss treatment with children, even teenagers. There were operations to place pins in his hip, one side at a time three weeks apart. The admission was long as walking was not allowed for three months and even getting around in a wheelchair was not enough to justify discharge. Nowadays, children with a slipped epiphysis are usually in hospital for only one week. There were school lessons every day, and one teacher supported children from elementary, junior high school and high school levels just like a country school. David's grades in grade ten were excellent, due to a combination of good teaching and the absence of social distractions to interfere with homework and school projects.

David has other memories. Like the others, he remembers the strict rule that all children had to get dressed, and pyjamas were not allowed by day. When hospital clothes were worn, the children were given some choices by the nurses. David remarked that some of the nurses who cared for him still work at ACH. He was in a four-bed room with a view of the city. To get dessert, he had to eat everything but one thing on his plate, but in fact some of the children put their discarded food onto one plate, and threw it out the window in winter. In the spring, once the snow melted, all the food was found, and the maintenance man and gardener (George Higbee) made the boys clean it up themselves. David joined the staff of the Alberta Children's Hospital in 1985. When he met George, he was still too embarrassed to remind him of this episode.

There were always other activities with crafts on Monday, Scouts on Tuesday, spiritual singing on Wednesday, Thursday evening was a quiet evening, but on Friday there were movies, and on Saturday there might be more movies or a drive in the handi-bus. Children were able to go to a church service on Sunday.

The ward was traditional, and the whole place looked and smelled like a hospital. However, David had been in an adult ward in Lethbridge and appreciated the advantages of a paediatric hospital, though the only contact he had with peers was with the other orthopaedic patients.

The orthopaedic residents were around much of the time, unlike the staff surgeons, and made a special effort to cultivate his early interests in medicine by sharing some of their medical textbooks with him.

Unquestionably, his positive experiences at the Alberta Children's Hospital proved to be influential to his decision to become a physician and paediatrician.

David graduated from The University of Calgary in Engineering and then returned to The University of Calgary to train in Medicine and is now on staff at the Alberta Children's Hospital as an endocrinologist.

PART FIVE

PREPARATION FOR A NEW ERA 1972−1981

❖❖❖❖❖❖❖❖❖❖❖❖❖

Developments in Health Care

The Government of the Province of Alberta became the owner of the Alberta Children's Hospital in 1972. This transfer of owner ship from the Alberta Children's Hospital Society was mutually beneficial for the government and the children of Calgary and southern Alberta. The government obtained a hospital which had a good reputation in the community and would help it to fulfill its mandate of delivering high-quality health care. The children, represented by the Alberta Children's Hospital Society, would benefit from the proceeds from the sale, which were placed in trust and used for services beyond those provided by the government. The Alberta Children's Hospital Society initially acted only as trustee for the investments from the sale of the hospital but later became an active fundraising organization as the Alberta Children's Hospital Foundation.

The Lougheed Government (which had been elected in 1971) was enthusiastic about this purchase of the Alberta Children's Hospital. There were some technical delays, as amendments to the various acts had to be introduced to allow for a second provincial hospital in Calgary.[1] The Foothills Hospital became a provincial hospital in 1966 as the Minister of Health wanted to make sure it was not controlled by either the University or the municipality. The paediatric unit in Foothills Hospital throughout the 1970s would develop considerable expertise and skill and be recognized as the centre for acute tertiary care services for children. The purchase of the Alberta Children's Hospital was in keeping with the trend established by the federal *Medical Care Act* of 1966. As part of the new approach to health care in Canada, the Government of the Province of Alberta had been paying about $1 million annually toward the running of the Alberta Children's Hospital. Both the government grants and the cost of running the hospital had risen steadily. In 1962, the total operating cost was $649,804.75 and the government grant was $524,099. By 1971, these figures had risen to $1,187,274.15 and $994,827.20 respectively.[2]

The Government Hospital Commission, as the new owner, appointed a Board which was responsible for the day-to-day operation of the hospital. This first board included a number of individuals who had been on the Alberta Children's Hospital Society Board and thus had experience in running a children's hospital, but there were new appointees and some individuals from the community.[3]

The appointment of an administrator responsible for the hospital was a major responsibility of the new Board. The successful candidate was Robert Innes, who had experience in acute care (Hospital for Sick Children in Toronto) and chronic care (Texas) and a strong vision of family-centred care. He played an extremely important role in the further development of paediatrics in Calgary.

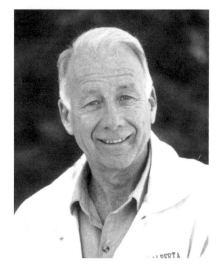

Bob Innes.

The expansion of a children's hospital at this time seemed very appropriate, as there were many more children than ever before. Not only were there more births, but children were now likely to survive to adult life. There was a sharp fall in deaths in childhood, and after the age of one year, death in childhood became uncommon. There were fewer stillbirths, and not many babies dying in the first year of life, compared with the early years of the century. There were many reasons for this falling death rate. In the 1920s and 1930s, most of the childhood deaths were due to infectious diseases. By 1972, this was only ten percent. Many lethal diseases had virtually disappeared, including diphtheria and polio, or were rare, such as tuberculosis. Other disorders (such as scarlet fever and streptococcal throat infection) were not only much less common, but also seemed to be less severe. Some illnesses occurred in periodic epidemics, but even these showed a remarkable drop in incidence, one example being pertussis. The reasons for the disappearance of the infectious diseases are complex. It is not simply a result of immunization, although this remains important, and has little to do with medical and nursing care and virtually nothing to do with the recently introduced government health schemes. Rather this improvement in the outlook for children had much more to do with a general improvement in nutritional standards, improvement in hygiene and was related to the overall economic well being of the country. Patterns of disease change and infectious diseases may become prominent again as a cause of death in childhood.

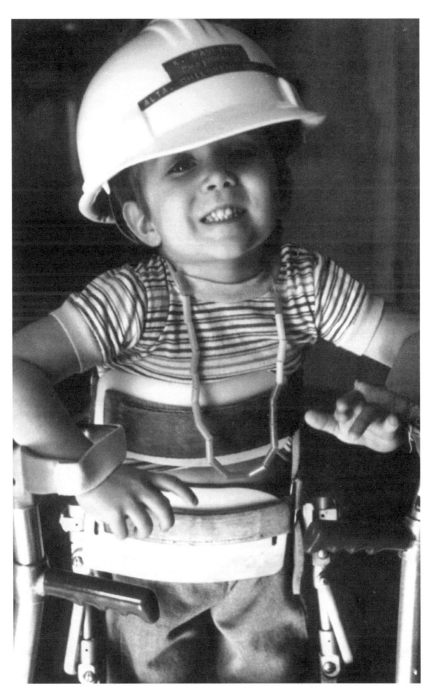

Happy and determined child.

The number of health-care professionals had increased much more than the population had increased throughout the twentieth century, and the number of individual professions had also increased dramatically.

	Physicians			Nurses	
	Numbers	**Population /Physician**	**Graduates of Canadian Medical Schools**	**Number**	**Population /Nurse**
1921	8,706	1,008	406	21,385	410
1972	34,508	636	1,280	156,630	140

Between 1921 and 1972, the dramatic increase in the ratio of physicians to population as a whole can be clearly seen,[4] similar to a large increase in the number of nurses and a change in the ratio of nurses to the population as a whole. This was supported by an increase in the number of medical schools from nine in 1925 to sixteen in 1970. The University of Calgary Medical School was one of the new medical schools, and remains the youngest of the Canadian medical schools with the first class graduating in 1973. Canada, despite these medical schools, was still dependent on immigrants who represented 43.5 percent of new physicians licensed in 1972. Nurses and physicians were joined by many members of new professions, such as physiotherapists, occupational therapists, speech therapists, psychologists, social workers and so on. Some of these practices, such as physiotherapy or orthoptics, started in the nursing profession and, with additional training, evolved into a separate profession. Formal training for these professions was provided in colleges and universities, and all the professions were represented at the Alberta Children's Hospital.

The priorities of paediatric care were changing dramatically. Children with acute illnesses, including acute infectious illnesses, still merited the best possible care, but previously unrecognized and under-recognized problems were now getting attention. These chronic conditions included illnesses such as diabetes, joint disease, chronic neurological diseases such as epilepsy, respiratory diseases such as asthma and also long-term consequences of illnesses such as polio. In addition, many infants who survived the newborn period after prematurity had a recognized handicap. All of these problems needed a systematic approach to the problems of the child and family over many years. Only by using such a systematic approach could a good result be obtained. This way of approaching old problems was called the "New Paediatrics," and paediatricians and other health-care providers wanted to be responsive to the needs of the child and family over many years, helping them deal with disease in response to changes in life circumstances and helping the child to grow and mature despite the presence of a chronic disease.

> *We begin with the premise that the needs of the chronically ill child cannot be met adequately in a system orientated toward the care of children with acute, episodic disorders or toward the supervision of those who are essentially healthy. Chronically ill children require care that is truly comprehensive, well coordinated and continuous. Comprehensiveness in this context involves an equal commitment to "management" as to "treatment"; this in turn implies an orientation to the whole child in the context of his family and its culture.[5]*

The philosophy behind the New Paediatrics was readily accepted at the Alberta Children's Hospital. Children with long-term orthopaedic problems had been given skilled and loving care for years, and it was easy to extend this to children with other chronic diseases. There was considerable pressure to develop the hospital into a child health centre, and the Minister of Health and Social Development (Neil Crawford) in the new Progressive Conservative government, encouraged the Advisory Committee for the Multiple Handicapped to continue its deliberations. This committee made its report in 1972 and recommended a child health centre.❖

References

1. *The Calgary Herald*, March 23, 1972.
2. *Annual Report*. Alberta Children's Hospital Society, 1962 and 1971.
3. First Board: E.F. Allison, W.R. Boswell, G.C. Johnson, K.M. Manning (Chairman), J.C. Orman, W.H. Tye.
4. Leacy, F.H., ed. *Historical Statistics of Canada*. 2nd ed. Statistics Canada, Table B82-92.
5. Pless, I.B., and K.J. Roghmann. "Chronic illness and its consequences: Observations based on three epidemiological surveys." *Journal of Pediatrics*, 79 (1971):351–359.

Plans for a New Child Health Centre

The Child Health Centre did not become fully functioning until 1982 when the Emergency Department opened and the care of acutely ill children, including those in the Intensive Care Unit, was transferred from the Foothills Hospital. The completion of the Child Health Centre was the successful result of a decade of planning, associated with hectic and at times acrimonious, political activity. Ten years earlier, the DAT Centre started with clinics in trailers, followed by the Dr. Gordon Townsend School (1977). It is difficult to pinpoint the exact origin of the idea of a Child Health Centre, but there is no doubt that parents were an extremely important driving force. Many of the parents involved, including a group called "Parents for Progress," wished a "new deal" for handicapped children. They were supported by paediatricians who had had training and experience in children's hospitals elsewhere and felt that infants and children in Calgary with severe acute and chronic handicapping illnesses should have all the benefits of a children's hospital as in other cities. Many other individuals, organizations and institutions played a role in planning for the Child Health Centre, and some changed their attitude more than once during the planning period. The hospital boards, particularly those in Calgary with paediatric units (Foothills, Calgary General and Holy Cross Hospitals) and The University of Calgary Faculty of Medicine played a major role. Some professional organizations such as the Alberta Paediatric Society, prepared detailed proposals for the Child Health Centre and endorsed the overall concepts.[1]

The provincial Department of Health had the final say about the Child Health Centre. One of the prime aims of the Lougheed Government, elected in 1971, was "delivering increased assistance to handicapped children."[2] The new government received the Report of the Advisory Committee for the Multiple Handicapped Program on July 1972, recommending a Child Health Centre.[3] The planned centre was to provide a co-ordinated, multidisciplinary approach for children with complex health, medical, mental, emotional and social problems and was to recommend appropriate programs to meet the needs. The Chair of the committee, Dr. Ian Burgess, a paediatrician in Calgary since 1969, was familiar with the level and pattern of care provided in the Children's Hospital in Winnipeg and was enthusiastic about opportunities in Calgary. All the committee members were involved in some aspect of child health and brought diverse backgrounds and points of view to the discussion and deliberations. The presence of acute care, chronic care and ambulatory care at one site was the preferred option of the committee.

Recommendations of the Diagnostic Assessment and Treatment Centre Task Force of Calgary of the Regional Mental Health Planning Council to develop a Diagnostic, Assessment and Treatment (DAT) Centre to provide a co-ordinated multidisciplinary approach to specific problems of childhood were in keeping with the view of the Burgess Committee.

Some of the work of the committee was important, but of little direct interest to the parents or the public. For example, one subcommittee reviewing laboratory services felt that none of the laboratories then available in Calgary specialized in micromethods (analyses on small samples, important in paediatrics) and that a larger laboratory at the Alberta Children's Hospital would meet this need without duplicating services. The X-ray Department at the Alberta Children's Hospital consisted of one small room, equipment which was twenty-two years old and a generator which was too low-powered for accuracy and clarity. A detailed proposal for a modern radiology department was developed by another subgroup. This plan included space for ultrasound, even then recognized as important in paediatrics as it provided images of the child without radiation. This focus on the child's safety would lead to the title "Diagnostic Imaging Department" to illustrate that radiation was only one of the modalities used. When conventional X-ray pictures of the child were taken, safety was emphasized by using a dose of radiation much lower than in other hospitals, something which still happens today.[4]

Acute care was to be provided at the Child Health Centre along with other components of paediatric care, but it would not be the only hospital in Calgary where acutely ill children could be admitted. The other three general hospitals would still have paediatric units. The report stated that:

A Child Health Centre would manage only those problems requiring neonatal intensive care facilities and those children requiring care for complex, acute illnesses... A very rough guess was made that the upper limit of approximately 25% of hospitalized children or less would need the specialized services of a Child Health Centre.[5]

Moreover, some services such as those for cardiovascular and renal diseases, conditions where there is a joint approach to paediatric and adult cases, were considered too expensive to move from the Foothills site at that time. By 1997, most tertiary paediatric services are provided at the Alberta Children's Hospital site, including services for children with cardiovascular and renal diseases, but neonatal intensive care services remain at Foothills Hospital, appropriately adjacent to the high-risk maternity unit.

Various sites were proposed for the Child Health Centre, and the issue of site, which had first been raised in 1966, continued to be contentious. The main choices were still between the Health Sciences site (adjacent to the Medical School and the new Foothills Hospital) and the traditional 17th Avenue site. Location of the Alberta Children's Hospital on the site of the Health Sciences Centre, adjacent to the Foothills Hospital, had some advantages, but there was concern that the needs of children on that site might not be fully met unless there was a board specifically responsible for the Alberta Children's Hospital and thus for paediatric issues. The Alberta Children's Hospital Board preferred the new Child Health Centre to be on the site they already owned on 17th Avenue, but were willing to move to the Foothills Hospital site.[6] On the other hand, the Foothills Hospital Board took the position that only one board could administer hospitals on that site, and therefore that it should be responsible for the Alberta Children's Hospital. The Burgess Committee was concerned that a board looking after such a large hospital as the Foothills would have insufficient time or interest to deal with the specific concerns of children and so, by a vote of eleven to four, the committee recommended "that the Child Health Centre be located at the Alberta Children's Hospital."[7] The final report of the Advisory Committee for the Multiple Handicapped Program was endorsed by the Minister of Health and also by the Chairman of the Alberta Children's Hospital Society, although the decision on the site was not confirmed by the government until 1974.[8]

The dispute over site was partly a dispute over leadership in paediatric health care. Was this hospital to be supervised by a large board with many competing responsibilities, or did the needs of children necessitate a separate organization? The issues had been described by Dr. G. Holman in his report in 1969. The dispute became bitter and personal, and Dr. G. Holman was forced to resign and left Calgary. He had proposed the Health Sciences site for the Alberta Children's Hospital but spoke out publicly in favor of a separate board for the Alberta Children's Hospital.[9] This was strongly opposed by the Foothills Hospital Board who supported only a few of the recommendations of the report. Many parents and paediatric professionals feared that a "Glenrose-type" solution would be imposed. This referred to an Edmonton hospital which had (and has) beds for children with mental health problems, an assessment centre for children with developmental delay and habilitation and rehabilitation services for children. It did not have beds for paediatric acute care, which were at all the other hospitals, although mainly at the Royal Alexandra Hospital and the University Hospital. The Glenrose also has extensive adult (including geriatric) rehabilitation services. Whether the publicity surrounding Dr. Holman's resignation, and the obvious professional and parental support for his point of view, played any role in the government's support cannot be known with certainty.

Later in 1974, Dr. R.H.A. Haslam was appointed Head of the Department of Paediatrics at The University of Calgary, following a short period when Dr. R. McArthur was Acting Director of Paediatrics. Dr. Haslam is a paediatric neurologist with a background in acute care and in chronic disease and was also appointed Head of Paediatrics at Foothills Hospital and at the Alberta Children's Hospital. From the moment of his appointment, he participated fully in planning and was invaluable in clarifying the issues for the boards concerned.

After a new Child Health Centre was approved by the Minister of Health, detailed planning began, and as summarized by Robert Innes,[10] this represented a major departure from previous methods. In the past when hospitals were being designed, there was a focus on the number of beds and emphasis on their layout and on planning of wards. Many felt that such a planning process, and its focus on beds, was not only inefficient but also insufficient to design a successful building. This would be a large contract, and so only a few architectural partnerships had enough resources to compete for the right to design the new health centre. Almost all of them relied on their previous experience in hospital design.[11] In contrast, the architects who were eventually selected (Cohos Evamy) were part of a large organization, but had the advantage of *no* previous experience in hospital design! Michael Evamy was the partner in charge of the project and was joined by Jim Goodwin, Bill Johnstone and Jim Hodges. This group began a broad conceptual planning analysis in April 1974 which included a detailed study to define community needs. Once it was established how many children were affected by a particular problem, the resources required could be identified. This process was time-consuming and involved community and staff. Once again a group from Calgary visited many other centres, including the Children's Hospital at Stanford and Los Angeles Children's Hospital. These architects immersed themselves in the process and were so keen to understand the problems faced by the children that they rode around the hospital in wheelchairs and were pushed around in hospital beds complete with orthopaedic equipment.

One of the first meetings attended by Jim Goodwin (who is still involved with developments at the Alberta Children's Hospital) was in the DAT Centre with mothers and children. One child came over slowly to Jim, sat near him and started to play with a ball. To make life easier while he played, the boy took off his socks and shoes and as he did so his feet also came off! He played quite nonchalantly with his stumps exposed and illustrated clearly that he was a child first and had accepted his own body. This young lad knew nothing of adult concepts of normal or abnormal. This experience served to emphasize to Jim that all children are "normal" to themselves and their parents, and that this awareness should be incorporated in their planning.

As the plan for the Child Health Centre was horizontal and not high-rise, it occupied a large area of ground. The overall theme, whatever part of the complex was being considered, was ambulatory, and determined efforts were made to de-institutionalize care. An important early development was the concept of the Child Space, which was central, open and gave easy access to many areas of the hospital such as the DAT Centre,

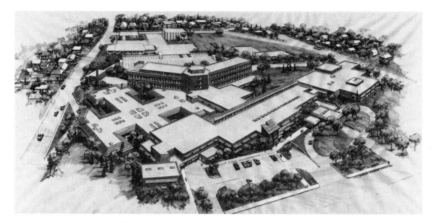

Architect's concept of the Child Health Centre.

school, in-patient clusters and cafeteria. Children going from the in-patient area to the school could choose their own route, as the architects provided a choice. Thus children living in the hospital had some of the freedoms that most children take for granted. The in-patient units were designed to encourage good communication and to reduce the "hospital atmosphere" while allowing for the child's developmental needs.

Care of the child and family can be affected by the organization itself, and thus lines of responsibility from an individual providing care at the Alberta Children's Hospital could go to the Board by different routes. There were parallels between the physical structure and the running of the Child Health Centre. For example, a child and family would receive care in one area from many different professionals, who would come to the child. These professionals worked together to offer the best service and achieve the best outcome and, as far as care was concerned, were responsible to the particular clinic director, whatever their discipline. However, for some issues, the professionals were also responsible to a department director of their specific discipline. This complex linkage of responsibility to different directors for different functions is called a "matrix" and works well if there is a spirit of co-operation and commitment to common goals.

Late in the planning process, the nurses at the Alberta Children's Hospital formed a Nursing Model Committee which met between February 1980 and May 1981 to address how nursing care might be provided in this unique hospital. The administrator of the in-patient division (B. Racine) used the Nursing Model Committee as a means to facilitate active staff participation in the planning of a nursing care system, and nurses from the existing nursing units were appointed to the committee. There were two head nurses and six staff nurses. This committee discussed a number of topics and developed a philosophy, including a concept of the role of the primary care nurse, ways in which patient care would be co-ordinated and how relationships and responsibilities would be developed. Protocols were designed, and the committee did simulations of work in the new part of the hospital. The committee eventually included new senior staff members with emergency and intensive care experience, as the original group were long-standing Alberta Children's Hospital staff members without such experience. There were no nurses from the acute unit at Foothills (or elsewhere in the city). This committee reflected on its role once it was completed and certainly felt that the involvement of staff nurses was a positive influence. In retrospect, they felt that the commit-tee should have been established at an early stage of planning and design and should have had closer links with the medical staff. Although the committee did not mention it in its own review, perhaps it would have been helpful to have built closer links with nurses who were being trans-ferred from the Foothills Hospital.

The school was the first part of the new construction to be completed and opened in 1977, two years before the foundations were laid for the DAT Centre and in-patient area. The school had been in temporary ac-commodations for some years, the teachers had made a formal com-plaint to the Calgary Board of Education through the Alberta Teachers' Association and closure of the school had been considered.[12] Once the Burgess Report was approved, priority was given to building the school to deal with the concerns of the teachers which related to such issues as fire safety, access to the school and lack of hot and cold running water. The plans for the school were scaled down from twelve classrooms to eight, but always included two pre-school rooms. At the design stage, it was intended that the enrollment would be children staying in the ACH, but this practice was changing rapidly as other schools became better able to cope with children with disabilities, and advances in medical care and availability of equipment allowed children to be more mobile.

The overall plan for the Child Health Centre, as initially developed, was to cost over $30 million. This was a far cry from the $5 million renovation suggested in 1973, with a completion date of October 1976. That small-scale renovation included minimal new building, but many internal changes to the 1952 building, including a paediatric intensive care unit on the fourth floor. However, to reach an agreement for the more extensive and expensive plan, there had been many meetings, and some of these were angry and bitter. The response to the initial cost estimates was a new round of meetings with the Alberta Hospital Serv-ices Commission. Many changes were made to reduce this cost, and all were approved by the Alberta Children's Hospital Board. For example, a hostel for parents was no longer included, and this need was partially met by the later construction of Ronald McDonald House (March 1985). Another cost saving was in the foundations. The original cost included

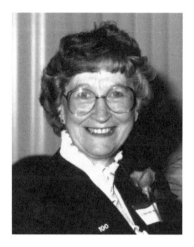

Dorothy Potts

with about thirty-four patients. After two years, she became the night supervisor with various jobs to do. One of them was going down to the boiler room to make sure the gentleman who looked after the boiler was still alive. At 4 a.m., she had to open the back door for the bread man and milk man and lock the door behind them again. At 6 a.m., the rotating toaster had to be turned on, and half an hour later all the doors were opened for the day shift.

D orothy was born on a farm in Lloydminster, Saskatchewan, in 1922. She was a teenager when the war broke out and really wanted to join. Instead she started her training in nursing in 1944, at a time when she had to pay for books, uniform and a tuition fee of about $20. Despite these drawbacks, two of her sisters also finished the School of Nursing. Dorothy also took a post-graduate course in operating techniques in Vancouver, and this knowledge helped her nurse post-operative patients. Later, as a teacher, she encouraged other nurses to learn about operating techniques early in training. She worked in Edmonton, Lethbridge and Victoria and, in 1958, arrived in Calgary to work in the Alberta Crippled Children's Hospital as a night nurse. Each night nurse was responsible for a floor, usually

In 1964, she succeeded Margaret Baxter as Director of Nursing. She strongly supported many important developments, such as changing visiting hours in 1965. Dorothy was actively involved in providing information to the Burgess Committee. She remained Director of Nursing until 1977, then became Director of Donations and Public Relations and was an outstanding success. She had a so-called retirement in 1989 but remains involved in hospital life. The preservation of many of the early records of the hospital is due to her interest in the history of the Alberta Children's Hospital.

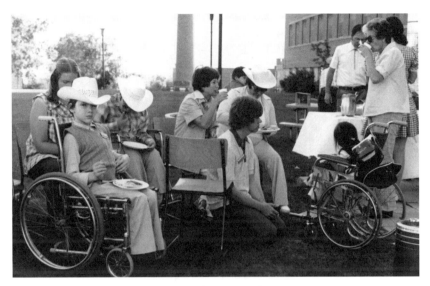

Stampede breakfast.

foundations which would be able to support a second level above in-patients should it ever be required, but these stronger (and more expensive) foundations were removed from the plans. Once the detailed plans[13] for the building were approved in 1975 as a $20 million project, foundations were laid[14] and, by October 1979, were completed.

However, planning the details of use of the new Child Health Centre continued long after the physical design was completed, partly because of the time that had already elapsed, but mainly because of the changes in paediatric practice throughout the Western world and in the organization of paediatric care in Calgary throughout the 1970s. The requirements of acute care began more and more to dominate the planning discussions. There was a financial windfall late in the process which allowed further development of acute care, albeit engendering further conflict with government. Federal sales tax (FST) was included in the purchase price of all building materials, but publicly funded works were entitled to a rebate, which was usually returned to the provincial government. The ACH "earned" a seven-figure rebate, which was used locally to increase laboratory space in the basement, extend the emergency department space to allow it to function beyond the urgent care level and provide "shell space" on the second floor which would be available for future development.

During these politically turbulent years, when so much time was spent ensuring that a world-class Child Health Centre would become a reality, the children were not forgotten and life in the hospital went on as before. Children were admitted and discharged and, while in hospital, received

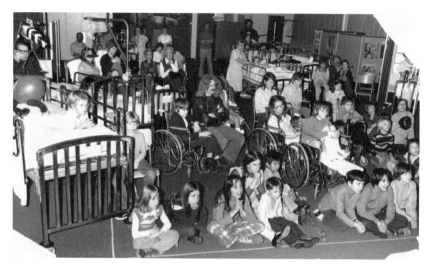

Fun in the solarium.

dedicated care from professionals who became part of their life. Children were involved in projects, such as the design of a Christmas card for 1973. There were no prizes, but many excellent ideas, and this project continued for several years.[15] The solarium was extensively used in the 1970s for activities, games and parties. There were outside activities, even for patients in plaster casts, and Stampede breakfasts continued. There were new initiatives; for example, the Junior League of Calgary opened and ran a toy library in the hospital. The toys were specifically aimed at developmentally challenged children and could help the children in many ways without cost to the parents.[16]

There were many specific developments in paediatric care in Calgary in the 1970s and most of them involved co-operation between the various hospitals and The University of Calgary. Some of the new services were placed in the Alberta Children's Hospital, but more were based at Foothills Hospital and were associated with the recruitment of specialist academic physicians. The changes which did occur in the in-patient unit at the Foothills Hospital are properly also part of the Alberta Children's Hospital history, as the workload of this unit and staff eventually transferred to the expanded Alberta Children's Hospital. The Foothills Board was supportive of its paediatric unit, as it developed a role in tertiary care over the years after the opening of the Foothills Hospital (1966) and the Medical School (1970). The physical layout of this paediatric unit was altered more than once to make it more appropriate for the care of children, and late in the 1970s there was a five-bed ward for oncology and a small school room.[17] The Paediatric Intensive Care Unit (PICU) opened in March 1979 with five acute and four progressive beds, and the Head

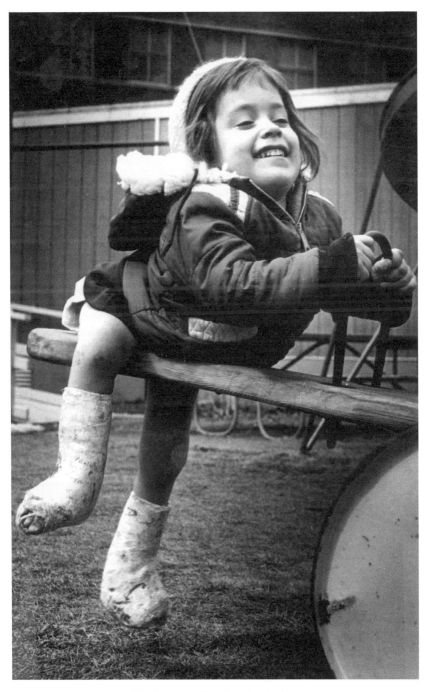

Playing on the teeter-totter.

Nurse (Nelda Harker) and Nurse Instructor (Phyllis Davis) continued in these roles in the Alberta Children's Hospital PICU when it opened in 1982. Medical supervision changed with time, reflecting developments in medical practice. At first, general paediatricians looked after their own patients in the PICU, later came general paediatricians with an interest in intensive care and, later still, paediatricians with specific training in intensive care. The first of these was Dr. D.M. (Gus) Cooper (also a respirologist) who became the Director of the Intensive Care Unit in 1981 and was able to participate in the choice of equipment in the new PICU at the Alberta Children's Hospital and in designing the new unit. He continued as Director of the Intensive Care Unit when it transferred to the Alberta Children's Hospital. Many subspecialty physicians were recruited jointly by Foothills Hospital and The University of Calgary Medical School in the decade before the Child Health Centre fully opened.

Along with developments in paediatric practice, there was a general interest in the re-organization of paediatric services within the City of Calgary and, in 1978, a committee representing the Child Health Centre, Foothills, Calgary General, Holy Cross and Rockyview hospitals was established to investigate the effect that the proposed changes in paediatric services might create among the various institutions. This group produced a position paper in April 1980 and among its recommendations was that the Child Health Centre be designated the tertiary care hospital for children in southern Alberta. The Calgary General, Foothills, Holy Cross and at a later date, Rockyview hospitals were to provide primary and secondary levels of care for children. The number of paediatric beds in each hospital was: Foothills, 68, with 75 percent occupancy; Holy Cross, 30–32 beds, with 62 percent occupancy; and Calgary General, 70 beds, with 55 percent occupancy.

There was far from unanimous support for the Child Health Centre (or even full understanding of the need), and one adult hospital administrator said that "often a child's illness is similar to the adult version, and our doctors in these cases are often more fully qualified and equipped."[18] Nevertheless a plea was made that all hospitals "co-ordinate activities wherever possible and together strive for the highest possible standards of child care."[19]

Some of the changes had more potential impact on Foothills Hospital than on the other hospitals, and therefore Foothills Hospital sought specific advice from its medical staff on future development. A subcommittee recommended that a unit for primary and secondary paediatric problems be maintained at the Foothills Hospital with the support of some "selected" tertiary services.[20] Some of this discussion leaked to the press, and politicians became involved. Dave Russell, the Minister of Health, pointed out that only children with more severe illnesses would come to the Alberta Children's Hospital, while children with milder illnesses would be admitted to other units in the city.

Meantime, more reasoned discussions were taking place in the background, and an external consulting firm was hired to work with the Foothills Hospital and the Child Health Centre to review all of the implications that reorganization of paediatric services might have on the two hospitals. The consultants arranged discussions between those involved in the provision of nursing care and medical services such as radiology, pathology and so on. On receipt of the report on the phasing-in process of the Child Health Centre, the Foothills Board again reviewed its role as far as paediatric services were concerned. By October 1980, the Foothills Hospital Board was seriously considering closing down all paediatric beds, maintaining only the Intensive Care Nursery. The Board passed this information to the medical staff which did not approve the recommendation. Despite this, at a meeting of the two boards and the Ministry of Hospitals and Medical Care on December 12, 1980, it was approved that over a period of two years, following the opening of the Child Health Centre, the Foothills Hospital would phase out its paediatric beds and services and transfer its paediatric caseload to the Child Health Centre. The Child Health Centre had a corresponding obligation to develop its facility to deal with these patients. It had to make provision for children in the Emergency Department and make specific arrangements for children requiring CT scanning, cardiac catheterization and renal dialysis, all three of which would still be provided at the Foothills Hospital site, even after the in-patient facilities were transferred. Nursing staff in paediatrics were to be given full consideration by the Child Health Centre for similar employment, and all medical staff at the Foothills Hospital who wished to apply would be given privileges at the Alberta Children's Hospital.[21]

Early in 1981, the announcement was made that the Foothills Hospital and the Alberta Children's Hospital had reached an agreement that in-patient care would be transferred to the Alberta Children's Hospital, which would also be the site for teaching paediatric care. This agreement was generally supported by paediatricians, but not by other physicians, particularly family physicians, who felt that the distance from northwest Calgary to the Alberta Children's Hospital was too far for parents to travel. There is no doubt that the episode generated many intense feelings, but attitudes were changing and the President of Foothills Hospital (R. Coombs) made a surprisingly prophetic statement that "Calgarians will get to know the Children's Hospital … as the place to seek care for their children."[22] ❖

References

1. Alberta Paediatric Society meeting, Red Deer, November 24-25, 1973.
2. *The Albertan*, March 3, 1972.
3. *Report of the Advisory Committee for the Multiple Handicapped Program*. Alberta Health and Social Development, July, 1972. Members of the committee were Dr. I.R. Burgess (Chairman), Dr. W.H. Mulloy, Dr. W.A. Cochrane, Dr. G.H. Holman, Dr.

N.C. Horne, Dr. N.T. McPhedran, Dr. M.G. Pearson, Dr. D.C. Blair, Dr. R.C.B. Corbett, Dr. R.G. Townsend, Mrs. R.M. Randall, Dr. C.H. Sangster, Frank Bach, Dr. P.B. Frost, Mrs. S. Sethi, Ken M. Manning, Martha Cohen, Mrs. Don West, R.L. Innes (Secretary).

4. *The Calgary Herald*, January 29, 1980.
5. *Report of the Advisory Committee for the Multiple Handicapped Program*, pp. 5 and 6.
6. *Minutes*. Alberta Children's Hospital Board, January 22, 1970.
7. *Report of the Advisory Committee for the Multiple Handicapped Program*.
8. *The Calgary Herald*, March 21, 1974.
9. *The Calgary Herald*, June 13, 1974.
10. Innes, R. Report of Interview, Chamber of Commerce, March 24, 1980.
11. Innes. R. Interview, November, 1996.
12. *The Calgary Herald*, March 27, 1974.
13. Proposal for Child Health Centre prepared by Alberta Children's Provincial General Hospital, September 30, 1974.
14. *The Calgary Herald*, June 20, 1975.
15. *The Albertan*, December 8, 1973.
16. *The Albertan*, December 2, 1976.
17. *Annual Report*. Department of Paediatrics, University of Calgary, 1978.
18. *Alberta Report*, March 21, 1980.
19. *Annual Report*. Department of Paediatrics, Foothills Hospital, 1980.
20. Paediatric Services Subcommittee, Medical Advisory Committee, Foothills Hospital, 1980.
21. *Annual Report*. Department of Paediatrics, Foothills Hospital, 1980.
22. *The Calgary Herald*, January 17, 1981.

Diagnostic, Assessment and Treatment (DAT) Centre

Children with long-term or lifelong complex handicapping illnesses have been a major focus for the Alberta Children's Hospital throughout its history. At first, these children were followed by private physicians only, but later it became clear that a team approach gave a better outcome. This concept developed rapidly and was part of the New Paediatrics. Such a team might include physicians from more than one specialty as well as the family physician/paediatrician and certainly included individuals from other professions such as physiotherapy, but with specific training in paediatric aspects. The Alberta Children's Hospital was not alone in the use of teams, a trend observed at many centres.

The centre in Calgary is rarely given its full name and is known simply as "DAT." Its objective has always been to provide comprehensive, co-ordinated and continuous care for children with complex health problems in Calgary and southern Alberta. The DAT Centre has been providing ambulatory care, which is another way of saying that overall care for the child is provided by the parents, who come to the hospital or Child Health Centre, from time to time, to receive help and advice in specific areas from professionals.

There would be "one-stop shopping" with the availability of specific expertise in many medical specialties and from many different professionals. The advantage of this centralized assessment centre was that parents did not need to travel to different sites throughout the city or even to different towns in the province to get an overall assessment of their child's many different problems. This comprehensive and centralized assessment process is coupled with a decentralized program of continuing care and support within the family and community with the development of appropriate services. The clinics were the focal point of the care of children and remain so, even when much of their care is received elsewhere, such as in the Preschool Treatment Program, ACH school, their own community school or as in-patients at the Alberta Children's Hospital. Children were to be assessed in their own clinic, and each clinic established appropriate links with public health units, other health-care facilities, day-care facilities and other services for children with disabilities. Some use the analogy of a three-legged stool to describe the role of the DAT Centre in the overall Child Health Centre. The DAT Centre is one leg, the treatment program another leg, and the in-patient program the third leg. The challenge is to keep the stool balanced, so that it can be used effectively.

The concepts and objectives of the DAT Centre preceded by many years its formal founding in 1972. Many clinics have been associated with the Alberta Children's Hospital over the years. Each one tended to work independently without formal structure or a common approach. For example, children with orthopaedic disorders had been seen at the hospital as out-patients from the beginning in 1922, before the orthopaedic out-patient clinic was formally recognized in 1935. By 1964, there was a Dental Clinic for in-patients and a monthly Cleft Palate Diagnostic Clinic with eight specialists in attendance. There was also a Speech Therapy and Assessment Clinic and an Orthoptic Clinic that had two fully trained orthoptists who worked with children with eye-muscle imbalance. This particular clinic saw a small number of adults (as did a number of other clinics in the early years) until the 1980s and was combined with the Ophthalmology Clinic to form the Eye Clinic in 1994. The Clinic for Juvenile Amputees was established with the support of the government and was given the go-ahead by the Board of Directors in 1964. Dr. J. Bazant directed the clinic, and the first one was held on December 9, 1965. Prostheses were prescribed and provided free of charge. The Orthodontic Clinic started at the end of 1965 as a free monthly service in co-operation with the Red Cross Society. A Preschool Hearing Clinic had been established in 1963, when the children affected were seen by a team of specialists, including an ENT specialist, paediatrician, speech therapist and social worker. This team completed a diagnostic and assessment of the child, then planned treatment and a home-care program for the parents. In 1969, a program was started for the in-patient care of emotionally disturbed children.

The Cerebral Palsy Clinic is one of the best examples of an early multidisciplinary clinic, which functioned quite independently of the Alberta Children's Hospital. In 1951, Dr. M. Cody sent a proposal to Colonel D.L. Tomlinson, Commissioner of the Alberta Division of the Red Cross, to have cerebral palsy patients seen at the Alberta Children's Hospital, either in the out-patient clinic or through admission.[1] His letter states, "we have had several cases where it has been proven that the treatment given has been most successful." The proposal was not accepted, and the first Cerebral Palsy Clinic was started at SAIT in 1956, initially with Dr. E.H.J. Smythe, then Dr. T.A. Richardson, and later Dr. A. Cody and Dr. Margaret Pearson.

Cerebral palsy was described by Dr. W.J. Little early in the nineteenth century and in more detail in the second half of the twentieth century by Dr. William Osler, the famous Canadian physician, and Dr. Sigmund Freud, who later became much more famous as a psychiatrist/psychoanalyst. Cerebral palsy is the result of damage to the immature brain. The damage occurs at one time (e.g., during pregnancy or at birth) and is not progressive, but its manifestations change as the child grows and develops. Cerebral palsy is a disorder of movement with many different types, the most common of which is spastic.

The medical facts, however, tell only part of the story. Cerebral palsy has a tremendous impact on the children themselves and on their families.

When the clinic was first started, there was no support system or access to appropriate education, and so the parents felt that there should be one centre devoted to the needs of their children. In September 1951,[2] the newspaper mentioned an out-patient clinic where treatment was provided to the "city's affected kiddies." There was some government support in the form of an occupational therapist and a secretary, but much of the help was provided by volunteers. For example, a fireman would pick up the children at home, take them to the playroom and return them home. Over the next few years, support staff were employed and more extensive services provided.

The managers of the Cerebral Palsy Clinic needed to find another location with the impending expansion at SAIT. As there was government support for the clinic, both the parents and the government agreed with the relocation of the CP Clinic to the Alberta Children's Hospital, which occurred in 1972 and was the first stage in implementation of the recommendations of the Burgess Report. This was a major move, with one hundred out-patients and support staff of twenty-six coming to the Alberta Children's Hospital or, more precisely, to eight portable trailers on the grounds. A tremendous effort was made to integrate the staff into the hospital, which until the transfer had had no occupational therapists, social workers or psychologists and only limited numbers of physiotherapists and speech and hearing experts. The CP Clinic expanded to include children with other conditions such as spina bifida (myelomeningocele) and muscular dystrophy. Thus the clinic was called the Neuromuscular Clinic in 1973, but many subdivisions of this clinic followed over the years, the first being the Myelomeningocele (Spina Bifida) Clinic in 1976. The CP Clinic continues today, under the name Neuromotor Clinic.

Further developments of the DAT Centre came with the appointment of medical directors and nursing leadership. The medical directorship was provided initially by Dr. Jack Brummitt who was Acting Director until 1974 and had worked in multidisciplinary clinics in Vancouver with Dr. Geoff Robinson. The first full-time director, and the first full-time physician on the Alberta Children's Hospital site, was Dr. Joe Moghadam who came from Toronto with experience in ambulatory care and public health. Other physicians were involved in the clinics but came from their private offices or from offices in other hospitals. Nursing leadership was provided by Andree De Filippi, who came to the Alberta Children's Hospital with the CP Clinic.

The Developmental Clinic was established in 1973 to provide services to children with mental retardation, emotional problems or learning disabilities and continues today. In the same year, the Asthma Clinic was designed to provide care for the small number of children with severe chronic asthma. The Cystic Fibrosis Clinic was transferred to the DAT Centre in 1973. This clinic had been started in the Calgary General Hospital

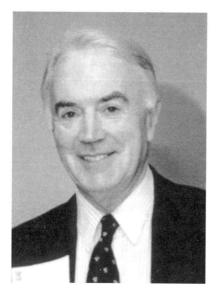

Brian Lowry.

by Dr. Richard Corbett in 1962 and initially acted as a consultant clinic to local physicians, but later evolved into a multidisciplinary clinic. At the time of transfer of the clinic to the Alberta Children's Hospital, comprehensive care could not be given, as in-patient care was inadequate for sick children. If admission was needed, it was to the Foothills, Calgary General or Holy Cross hospitals. By 1982, the Cystic Fibrosis Clinic in the DAT Centre was supported by the clusters for those needing admission, and a research program started. The Asthma and Cystic Fibrosis clinics continue as part of the Respiratory Service.

The Genetic Clinic was started in 1975 by Dr. Ian Burgess who combined a general paediatric practice with an interest in genetics. This clinic and service developed much more fully when Dr. Brian Lowry was recruited from the University of British Columbia to head the genetics group in 1977. Dr. Lowry already had national recognition, and under his leadership the Genetic Clinic became part of the Provincial Hereditary Disease Program.

There were other clinics under the general leadership of the DAT Centre but not all were on the Alberta Children's Hospital site. For example, the clinic for children with diabetes and endocrine disorders was at Foothills Hospital with Dr. Robert McArthur as Director and a nurse coordinator and only later moved to the Alberta Children's Hospital. When Dr. R.H.A. Haslam became Head of Paediatrics, he started a Neurology Clinic at the Alberta Children's Hospital site and later recruited Dr. Hussam Darwish and subsequently Dr. Harvey Sarnat to join him, as they further developed neurological services. Other clinics that developed in the 1970s were the Child Abuse and Family Resource Program (1977), Juvenile Arthritis Clinic (1976), and Hemophilia Clinic (1977) (for children and adults, even today). The Perinatal Follow-up Clinic, started in 1977 by Dr. Reg Sauve, who remains its Director, is an example of co-operation between the Intensive Care Nursery (now known as the Neonatal Intensive Care Unit) at Foothills Hospital and the Alberta Children's Hospital and provides follow-up and thus detailed information on the outcome of neonatal intensive care. More recently, there has been collaboration between these follow-up services and similar ones in Edmonton.

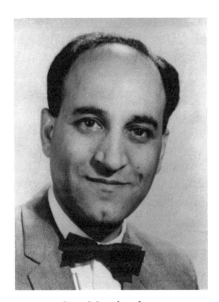

Joe Moghadam.

Many of the clinics pursued a common format. There was a director (usually a physician but not always), a co-ordinator (almost always a nurse) and a team of specialists from many different health professions. The strategy of the DAT administration in the early stages was to encourage as many clinics as possible to open when the new hospital was being constructed. It was felt that once the hospital was complete, the demands of the acute care unit, including the ICU, Emergency Department and operating rooms, would make it difficult to obtain resources for ambulatory care. Thus, by 1975, there were thirteen clinics; by 1977, sixteen clinics; and by 1983, thirty-one clinics serving the children of southern Alberta and their families. While this strategy was successful in developing the DAT Centre, the use of a standard staffing format for each clinic and the large number of clinics themselves were seen by others as wasteful and not a good use of resources.

The care provided in the hospital or DAT Centre can only be effective with liaison between the hospital and community. Dr. Moghadam, who had experience in ambulatory care and public health, was instrumental in working with Calgary Health Services to have a community health nurse at the Alberta Children's Hospital. The first such community health nurse (Eva Marvin) was appointed in January 1975 to act as a liaison between the DAT program and public health units in the city and rural areas. She provided first-hand input to DAT staff on the child and his/her family and also worked with community agencies to help them understand and follow through on recommendations made in the DAT Centre. Shortly afterward, Eva Marvin took a role as nurse co-ordinator in the Developmental Clinic and was succeeded as Public Health Liaison by Diane Ellingson in mid-1975. While the position no longer exists, the need for liaison remains important and still takes place at many formal and informal levels. Indeed, as children are now cared for at home with more complicated and severe problems than ever before, close contact with all home-care services is increasingly important. In this respect, the action taken by the DAT Centre to have a liaison between services at the hospital and public health agencies is a forerunner of what might be achieved by an effective regional health service.

Many facilities in Calgary provided therapy for the multihandicapped child, and the Alberta Children's Hospital was an enthusiastic partner with many of these organizations. One example was the Providence Child Development Centre (PCDC), which was managed by a joint committee, including Alberta Children's Hospital representatives, and had occupational therapy, physiotherapy, and speech therapy services provided and paid for by the Alberta Children's Hospital.

The Alberta Children's Hospital and DAT Centre developed a Community Advisory Committee composed of parents with a common concern for their handicapped child with a mission to bring together various support agencies within Calgary and southern Alberta to respond and listen to patients.[3] They had a major role in pointing out to health-care professionals, politicians and bureaucrats that the child is, and should remain, part of a community and not be isolated. The end result is that there was a strong desire for children to be kept at home as much as possible, while recognizing the great need of multihandicapped children and their supporting families; many programs had to be provided. The first suggestions and advocacy often came from the Advisory Committee. The document containing their recommendations has a drawing of many children on the cover which was used as a model for the quilt that hangs directly opposite the hospital's Admission area today.

The specific outreach programs developed by the Alberta Children's Hospital were in keeping with the general philosophy of working with parents and supportive of the work done by the public health liaison and other facilities such as PCDC. The first outreach program was supported by the visionary leadership of Robert Innes and developed by Ruth Cripps in 1972. Some of the outreach programs were developed because of the practical fact that there was insufficient room at the ACH site. Rather than putting up more temporary trailers, the Speech Pathology Department came up with an innovative solution. They decided to have a base at the hospital but to provide their services outside the hospital in local churches and community centres. At one point, there were sixteen mobile speech therapy teams, all part of one Speech and Hearing Department at ACH, directed by Caroline Dunsmore.

Other outreach programs developed following the example of the Speech and Hearing clinics, and all followed the youngsters with disabilities into the community to give extended therapy following a period of treatment and assessment at ACH. There were satellite programs, such as the mobile hearing vans which visited Lethbridge and Medicine Hat. The Orthoptics Clinic regularly visited Medicine Hat (and held its program on a stage in a large auditorium) with equipment housed in the "props" cupboard. The Genetics Clinic had outreach services in Lethbridge, Medicine Hat and Red Deer, and indeed still does today.

The Community Outreach Program had four different forms: direct work with the child, indirect care to the child with support for parents and teachers, assistance to communities to develop their own programs, and educational presentations to the public or professionals. The mobile teams were mostly used in Calgary, and these included a physiotherapist, occupational therapist and speech therapist, all placing major emphasis on the early integration of preschool children with disabilities. These teams still function today.

The Big Country Outreach Program, for the area around Drumheller, had international prominence, and Ruth Cripps was invited to other countries, such as Australia and Singapore, which had heard so much about this program in Calgary and southern Alberta and were in the process of starting programs as well. By 1990, many of the outreach services had been disbanded or had been taken over by many local communities or agencies, and the only one continuing is the Preschool Program.

Thus, the early DAT programs were provided in trailers on the ACH site, in many community sites and mobile teams. It was against this background that the architects started their planning for the physical layout of the DAT Centre, which had to be compatible with the overall philosophy of the hospital. The architects had many visits with professionals and with staff. Their combined vision was that the "patient unit" (in other words, child, parent and siblings) should attend a DAT clinic area. Once in a particular area, all assessments would be completed there without the child and family needing to move throughout the building. In other words, professionals were to come to the child rather than vice versa. The professionals were allocated personal offices on the second level of the Child Health Centre, but had to come to the clinic to provide treatment and assessment of children. These ideas triggered major opposition as most of the professionals wanted their own room in the DAT area. The new ideas were championed by Robert Innes and Dorothy Potts and held sway. In the early days, the areas within the DAT Centre were not allocated to specialties, but now all clinics have permanent designated areas.

Parent Services is an important program founded in 1973 by Nancy Watson, a volunteer in the Cerebral Palsy Clinic. This program recognizes that professionals cannot provide all of the care that children and families need, although great progress has been made following the visionary ideas of the early designers of the DAT Centre, by providing care for children in a space which allows enjoyment. Nevertheless, parents and children remain under considerable stress, and the friendly support and understanding provided by Parent Services in a non-judgmental manner is extremely important. These professionals are available, without appointment, at a highly visible point within the DAT Centre, ready to give parents directions to a clinic or service or extensive help in their dealings with physicians, therapists or clinics themselves. Families are

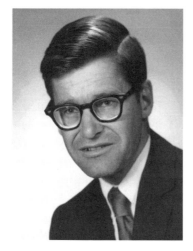

Ken Manning

The Board chaired by Ken Manning had members from many different backgrounds working together and actively involved in many aspects of planning and building the new Child Health Centre. There were many meetings with the community, deputy ministers and politicians to ensure that there was an open relationship with everyone aware of what was going on. It is a matter of great pride that the daily routine of the hospital went on as usual during major construction, with only minor interruptions.

Ken Manning was born and raised in Calgary and had contact with the Alberta Children's Hospital as a boy in 1936. His father, a Kinsman, took him along during his own volunteering for the hospital.

Later, he became general manager of his family lumber company, then started his own real estate firm. He himself joined the Kinsmen in 1956 and became chairman of their hospital committee. In 1959, he joined the newly formed Board of Directors of the Alberta Crippled Children's Hospital Society and remained a member until the province took the hospital over in 1972. He was not only a member of the first board appointed by the hospital, he was its first chairman and remained in that position until 1982.

One of his most enjoyable memories was the opening ceremony in 1981 when children were included and he participated in games and had a lot of fun. He had told Mr. Lougheed that the ceremony would be shared with those whom the hospital serves – the children! He still feels the hospital is a special *people place* with a warm atmosphere.

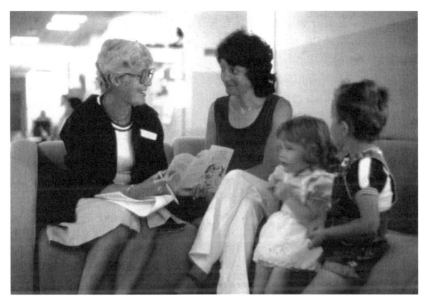

Nancy Watson in Parent Services.

always encouraged to participate knowledgeably in their own health care and to learn techniques of effective communication. Great efforts are made to foster an attitude that the family itself is the most important part of the health-care team and serves as an effective link with the hospital and community. Parent Services provides information on community services and support groups, in addition to its own important direct support.

There have been many changes in the DAT Centre over the years to accommodate various changes in medical practice and different needs of the hospital, but it remains an important segment of the overall Child Health Centre. Today, many services, such as Oncology, which are not strictly part of the DAT Centre, now work under the same multidisciplinary model, which has been accepted as the best way of caring for children with chronic disease. The strength of the Child Health Centre has always been the strength of the DAT Centre, and its close co-operation with all in-patient services.❖

References

1. Letter from Dr. M. Cody to Col. Tomlinson, June 19, 1951, p. 2.
2. *The Albertan*, September 19, 1951.
3. *The Calgary Herald*, September 22, 1973.

PART SIX

THE FOURTH HOSPITAL
1982–1997

❖❖❖❖❖❖❖❖❖❖❖❖❖

A New Beginning

T here are at least three dates that might be considered opening dates, each has a different significance and together they span a year from March 24, 1981, to April 1982.

The first opening ceremony was informal and fun. On March 24, in-patients who were in the old building were moved to the new building. They had been assigned their new rooms, and in fact there were only ten patients in the hospital that day. The children had already looked around the new rooms and moved some of their personal effects. The transfer

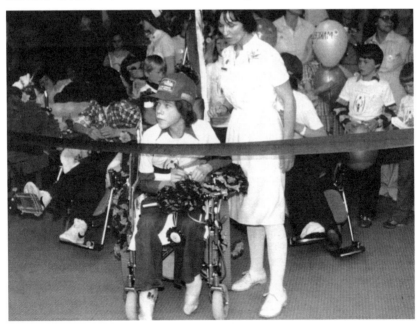

Unofficial opening.

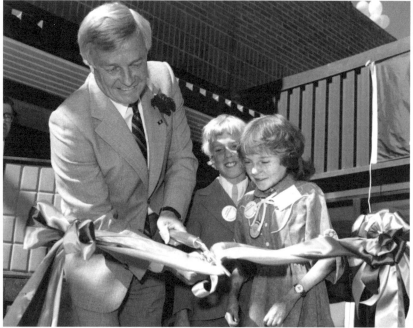

Photo courtesy of Argus Photography

Official opening.

took the form of a parade. The children had souvenir T-shirts and pins, their wheelchairs and beds were decorated with streamers and balloons, and there was a marching band, clowns, and "floats," all escorted by the RCMP. There were some fun speeches, a ribbon-cutting ceremony (performed by a child) and parties in the clusters.[1]

The second opening was the formal one on September 10, 1981. This was after the first transfer of children from the old hospital to the new one, but before all the facilities of the new hospital were ready.[2] The ceremony was performed by Premier Peter Lougheed and two children (Jennifer Collins and Michael Wilkinson) who represented all the children of Alberta. There was an embarrassing delay as it took many attempts to cut the ceremonial ribbon with the large scissors provided, but eventually the hospital was "officially" opened. These particular ceremonies were widely reported not only in Calgary, but also in local newspapers in the nearby towns of Lethbridge and Drumheller. Among the many dignitaries present was Mayor Ralph Klein, who commented that the hospital was "innovative, futuristic and sensitive to the needs of the children and parents."[3]

At the time of the official opening, a plaque was placed on the wall which summarizes the philosophy of the staff and Board of the Alberta Children's Hospital:

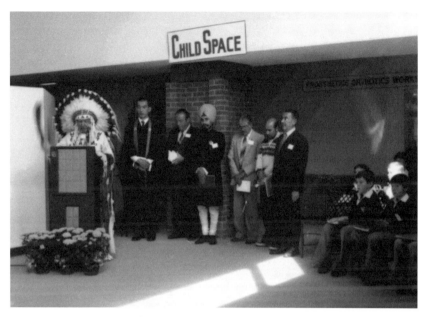

Blessing the new hospital.

*The Child Health Centre is dedicated to Alberta's most pre-
cious resource – our children – here, care extends to the spirit,
as well as to the body; the prevention of illness is fundamental; the regard for the family and the involvement of the community are foremost.*

On Sunday, September 13, there was an interfaith service to bless the
hospital and the people who worked there. This included a reading from
the Hebrew Bible, hymns and songs and, after a Christian blessing, bless-
ings from a Buddhist, a Hindu and a Muslim imam. To emphasize the
Canadian location of the hospital, the blessing by a Native Chief was
considered important.

The next day, there was a reunion of former patients and staff. People
had come from all over Alberta and British Columbia for this event. For
the staff to see "their" children again was wonderful, and many a story
and tear were shared. They almost had to share the buns and beef, because the two hundred people who attended had not been anticipated.

In the months after the official opening, other parts of the hospital
opened in a planned sequence. In January 1982, the Paediatric Intensive
Care Unit (PICU) opened, with the safe transfer of patients from Foothills
Hospital in freezing weather. Later, once all the facilities, including Operating Rooms, were functional, the Emergency Department opened; a child
could now be admitted to the Alberta Children's Hospital and given care no
matter how severe the illness. Thus the final step in the year-long opening

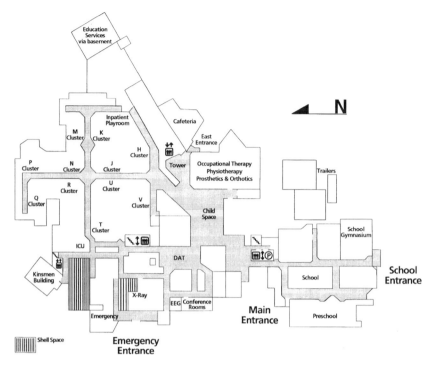

Main floor, 1982.

"ceremony" was public access to an Emergency Department devoted solely to children, which, in addition to providing medical and nursing assessment and treatment, also had a "hot line" for phone advice.

By 1982, a tour of the brand new hospital revealed many of the new facilities and impressive overall design. The main entrance can be approached from the street or by elevator from the parkade. The Dr. Gordon Townsend School can be entered from the hospital at this point, and in the other direction is the spacious Child Space and immediately beyond the Child Space on the west side the DAT Centre. The sketch shows the main divisions of the DAT area and how easy it is to move from the DAT area to various departments such as EEG or the X-ray Department. There is also an easy transition from the DAT area to the in-patient area. The in-patient units are called "clusters," which indicates both the variety of activities in a unit and also how these units relate to one another. Each cluster has a central area for parents and children, outside access to a courtyard and a direct entrance from the hallway into each room, which are mainly equipped with twin beds. The beds are at right angles, rather than the traditional parallel arrangement, allowing children to see one another. Each cluster has a small, narrow, galley entrance intended to have only such items as a fridge and some food storage. In the absence of

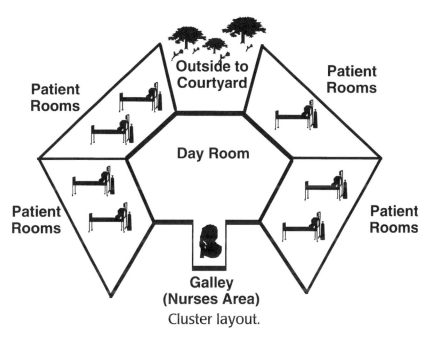

Patient Rooms

Outside to Courtyard

Patient Rooms

Day Room

Patient Rooms

Patient Rooms

Galley
(Nurses Area)

Cluster layout.

a dedicated area for physician/nurse charting and so on, the galley was soon taken over for this purpose, although cramped and unsuitable. This problem was not remedied until the twinning of the clusters in the late 1980s and early 1990s. The furniture was innovative and practical; its designer received a prestigious national award.[4]

Clusters were designated by age, rather than by medical or surgical specialty. This made sense from a child's point of view as, for example, the care needs of infants have much in common, whatever the diagnosis. Although many physicians and nurses opposed designation by age rather than by specialty, it was still implemented. Exceptions are required for highly technical care, Oncology, Orthopaedics, Mental Health and Intensive Care.

Carpets were used throughout the new building to give a "homey" look, but they were a source of inconvenience, and it is no surprise that there is difficulty in keeping them clean. There were poor facilities in each cluster for isolating children with infectious diseases, with a shortage of single rooms and an extreme shortage of sinks. Despite these problems, the open area for children and parents to be together was a major positive feature.

In the overall design, three areas important for sick children were geographically close together – the Intensive Care Unit, the Emergency Department and the Operating Room, and all three were near the X-ray Department and the DAT area. The Genetic Department and Behavioural Research Unit are in the Kinsmen Research Unit, which is not physically located in the hospital, yet still part of the Child Health Centre.

The floor plan on page 166 shows how easy it is to do a circular tour of the hospital from the DAT area, through the corridors around the in-patient units and then back to the DAT area from the other side. Other in-patient facilities on Level I included the cafeteria, workshop for Orthotics, physiotherapy pool and kitchen and dietary area. Overall, on an initial tour, the open design and lack of doors are noteworthy.

On Level II, there were important patient-care services for specific functions and personal offices for many professional staff. The patient-care functions on Level II were the Operating Rooms and the attached Dental Suite and Day Surgery. The offices for professional staff included the academic offices for the physicians who were members of The University of Calgary Department of Paediatrics and the other professionals including Psychology, Social Work and Speech Therapy, each with their own reception area.

There were many important departments in the basement of the new building, an area not usually visited by patients. These included all of the laboratories, such as Haematology, Biochemistry, Microbiology, Cyto-Genetics, Histology and the Autopsy Room. There was no Immunology Laboratory or Blood Bank, and the space designated for these was occupied by the Pulmonary Function Laboratory. The Pharmacy and Staff Health departments were also in the basement. A sloped corridor led up from the new basement to the basement of the 1952 building where Maintenance, Plant and Biomedical Services, important but often overlooked services, were located.

The old building is still used for many activities. The Ophthalmology Clinic, Child Abuse Department and Library are on the second floor. Office and treatment areas for many therapists are in one wing of the third floor and administrative offices and board rooms in the other wing. The lecture theatre is on the fourth floor and is still called the Solarium.

Some of the trailers stayed, providing temporary accommodation for the Alberta Children's Hospital Foundation. The old annex is still used as a nurse education area.

Overall, this new Child Health Centre was the embodiment of a grand concept which prevented the traditional and rigid separation of acute care, habilitation and rehabilitation and whose design and structure encouraged continuity of care. The development of the Child Health Centre had not been without problems and concerns, but its very design was evidence that they had been successfully surmounted, perhaps because of community input. During construction, there were strikes, occasional shortages of materials and some cost increases as Calgary itself was booming. The final cost was $40 million. Thus, the hospital was over budget and a year late in completion, not unreasonable given the magnitude of the task. One commentator actually commended the efficiency of all concerned in building the hospital so close to the cost estimate.[5]

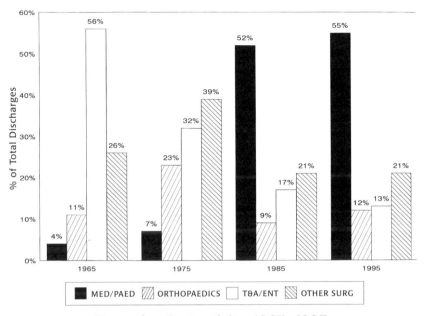

Type of patient activity, 1965–1995.

There remained some controversy even after the opening. For example, family physicians at the Foothills Hospital still felt that the Paediatric
Ward there was essential and warned that there would be dire consequences if the Paediatric Ward at the Foothills Hospital was closed. These
warnings seemed to come true in the fall of 1982, when a ten-year-old
girl attended the Emergency Department at the Foothills Hospital with a
broken leg, was transferred to the Alberta Children's Hospital, and, as there
were no beds at that hospital, then transferred to the Rockyview Hospital.
Ultimately, the child's fracture was reduced but only after many hours had
elapsed after her first attendance at an emergency department. There was
widespread publicity, but most observers saw this as an aberration from the
routine of high-quality care rather than a norm of poor or dangerous care.

For the first time in Calgary, one hospital had facilities for almost all of
the injuries and illnesses of childhood, although those which were common showed great changes from 1922 to 1982. The infant death rate in
Canada was low at 9.6 per 1,000 live births. Serious illness and death
were no longer a common experience, but paradoxically their low incidence strengthened expectations for a high level of care. Now efficient
care was provided for children with severe acute illness in the Intensive
Care Unit, the Operating Room, the Emergency Department and the
Clusters, and professionals recruited in the previous decade to The
University of Calgary and Foothills Hospital in paediatric sub-specialties
were an essential component in the provision of such care. The same

professionals were actively involved with children with chronic illnesses on the same site. The graph shows the illnesses treated at ACH in four time periods. Paediatric medicine was the largest single group in 1985 and 1995.

The community itself had changed rapidly in ways that were common in the Western World. Some developments were important to child care, such as the changing role of women and smaller family size. This is reflected in the fertility rate (a measure of the number of children by an individual woman), which had risen to 3.8 in 1960 at the height of the baby boom but fell to 1.8 in 1982. There were other changes, and though women were now much more likely to have their own careers and career aspirations, in child health, they continued to take a leadership role in many different ways, particularly if their own child had a health-care problem. In families with two children, it was likely that both parents worked outside the home. Single-parent families had become more common, usually headed by women. While some such families were affluent, many had marginal incomes, and a few exhibited evidence of extreme poverty, which in itself impacts on the incidence and severity of childhood disease.

To satisfy the demand for a high technical level of care, new equipment was acquired in 1981 for all areas. For example, Diagnostic Imaging acquired the second Emission Computed Tomography (ECT) scanner in the world (the first was in Los Angeles). This was described in news reports as "an inside-out X-ray machine," and feedback on its value was provided to the manufacturer, whether the patient was a premature newborn or a high-school football player.[6] There were many other examples of new equipment, the total cost of which was almost $10 million.

Support was provided to the hospital in many ways, one of which was fundraising. There were creative ideas; one, for example, came from the inmates at the Drumheller Penitentiary in 1983. Six inmates started out on foot on a 145-kilometre "con-walk" from Drumheller to Calgary, and through pledges and donations, an extensive amount of money was contributed.[7]

The staff in the hospital who deliver care are more important than the building or equipment. Hospital staff in 1981 and 1982 came from different backgrounds, and it is easy to discern at least three distinct groups. The first included staff specifically recruited for the new Child Health Centre, many from outside Calgary and a few from outside Canada. They were impressed with the new facilities, but as most of them had experience with children's hospitals elsewhere, they felt that the task of developing a tertiary level children's hospital was in its infancy.

The other two groups were the original Alberta Children's Hospital staff and the staff transferred from Foothills Hospital. The original Alberta Children's Hospital staff had skills in chronic disease and were delighted with the new building and its expanded facilities, but a little apprehensive about new areas and services such as the Intensive Care Unit and Emergency Department. The other group, the approximately thirty staff members who had been transferred from the Foothills Hospital, had experience with acute illness and were pleased with the new facilities but had mixed feelings about the move. These two groups, with their different skills, were both important to the success of the Child Health Centre but had little understanding or respect for one another. Such problems extended beyond the staff nurse level to a senior administrative level. Eventually the two groups developed respect for one another's skills and appreciation of the many different components that go into a Child Health Centre, but only after many years. Indeed, some believed that this mutual recognition was not achieved until the nurses' strike of 1988. It is interesting to note that of staff transferred from Foothills Hospital, twenty are still at the Alberta Children's Hospital in 1997.

Despite some problems, the new Child Health Centre was to prove a resounding success. All staff members, whether professional or support, were soon working together to provide the best possible care for the children and their families.

References

1. Nursing Model Committee, Alberta Children's Hospital, notes, p. 59.
2. *The Calgary Herald*, September 12, 1981.
3. *The Calgary Mirror*, September 15, 1981.
4. Government of Canada and the National Design Council 1983 Design Canada Award of Excellence.
5. *The Calgary Herald*, April 26, 1982.
6. *The Calgary Herald*, October 10, 1981.
7. *The Drumheller Mail*, June 23, 1983.

Programs in the 1980s and 1990s

The Child Health Centre opened with high hopes for the future and enthusiasm to develop the hospital. Staff were not fully confident of their ability to cope with a greater volume of children with acute illnesses, but time has proven that they can do so without losing their ability to focus on the needs of the whole child. Over the years, questions about the quality of service and whether the hospital is big enough or on the right site have led to several internal and external reviews. The most important was in 1987, when external consultants recommended expansion of the hospital to better meet the needs of children, and their suggestions were largely carried out. That committee also suggested relocation to the Foothills site. The second intensive review was in 1994, when again the issue of site was raised and it seemed as if the hospital would close. Developments in many departments through the 1980s and 1990s measure how much the dreams of the planners of the 1970s have become reality.

The most striking development since 1982 is the sheer number of children seen. In-patient discharges in 1971 were 3,172, of which 87 percent were surgical. By 1982, there were 4,817 discharges, and currently there are 6,000 per year, approximately fifty percent medical and fifty percent surgical.[1] The graph shows average number of discharges in five-year periods from 1965 to 1996.

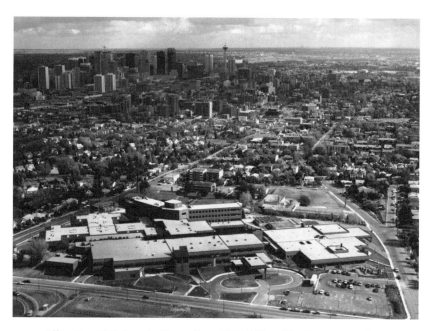

Alberta Children's Hospital Child Health Centre today.

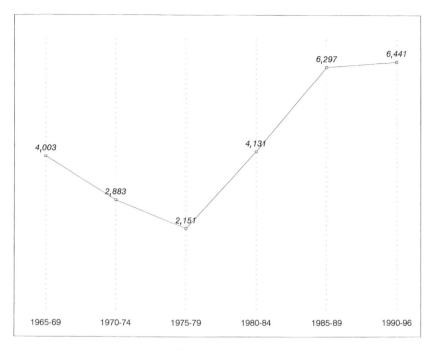

In-patient discharges, 1965–1995.

The attendance at Emergency increased dramatically; the numbers seen in first eleven months of operation (1982 to 1983) were 11,591, and are now just under 40,000 per year.

There was an increase in staff during the 1970s, and, by 1981, there were 552 employees. By 1982, this had risen sharply to 1,000 employees to accommodate the expansion.[2] In 1982, there were 210 physicians and seventeen dentists;[3] a moratorium on medical staff was declared on June 1, 1982.

When the hospital opened, the grant from the Department of Health increased sharply, and in the graph the low level of grants in 1972 ($1,494,765) and a sharp rise between 1980 ($13,297,555) and 1983 ($37,140,479) can be seen.[4] The government provided steady increases in funding, in keeping with the increase in workload and inflation. There was a further increase in 1989/90 to accommodate the opening of the extension at the front of the hospital and a sharp drop in 1994 as part of the cutbacks.

Calgary continues to have low use of in-patient beds compared with other cities in Canada as a result of the extensive ambulatory services supporting the home care of the sick child. These supports will require close scrutiny as health-care "reforms" and cutbacks evolve because many of the children who make extensive use of ACH have chronic diseases with disabilities in more than one system of the body. They have fared

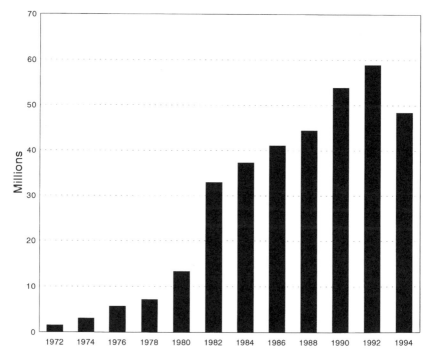

Department of Health grants, 1972–1995.

badly because they require services from education and social services as well as from health services, all of which have experienced severe cutbacks so that families experience them on more than one level.[5]

Nurses are the cornerstone of care at the Alberta Children's Hospital. The increase in the breadth and depth of nurses' skills reflects an increase in complexity of illnesses. Some of the reviews of nursing services have been important for all parts of the hospital, and some of the problems listed in the Nursing Department's own review eighteen months after opening are still unsolved in 1997. These include identifying the correct allocation of beds for psychiatry, deciding the type of care required for long-term patients, how to provide respite care and accommodation for parents to be in the hospital with their child.

One early problem affected both physicians and nurses, and this related to the number of beds. Only 116 beds were opened rather than the planned 128. The response of the administrators was to ask physicians to transfer patients to the vacant paediatric beds at the Holy Cross and Calgary General hospitals. Physicians however were unwilling to transfer patients and pressed for the Alberta Children's Hospital to become fully operational. This pressure on beds led to difficulty in maintaining age-related clusters so that, for example, a teenager and a baby might be in the same

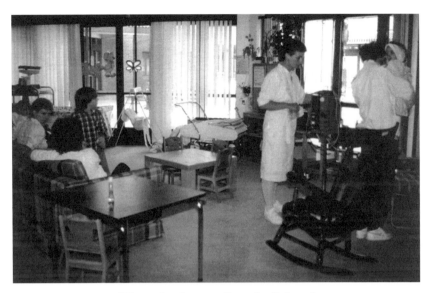

"There's always time to listen."

room from time to time. When a "better" placement was found for one or other of them, the problems were not over. For example, drugs were made up in specific dose amounts for a specific child and delivered to the patient's room. If the patient had moved in the meantime, there was potential for harm.

Of the many reports on ACH made between 1982 and 1997, the 1987 report commissioned by Calgary Area Hospital Advisory Council (Haggerty Committee) led to changes in service and to physical alterations in the hospital.[6] Four physicians from Canada and the U.S.A. (Dr. R. Haggerty, Dr. R. Goldbloom, Dr. E. Outerbridge and Dr. F. Guttman) conducted the review and were impressed with the dedication of staff at the Alberta Children's Hospital, the inclusion of allied health workers as members of the medical team, the outreach program and community involvement. There was general concern about the lack of medical input into Board decisions. More specific concerns were that, perhaps because of its background as a chronic disease hospital, the Alberta Children's Hospital had not developed some key acute care services, the number of beds was insufficient, and the hospital would be better placed on the Foothills site. The long-term impact of this review is illustrated by the fact that suggestions to improve ACH were all eventually carried out. These included an observation ward within the Emergency Department, opening of all the beds at the Alberta Children's Hospital, developing out-patient oncology and a cardiac catheterization laboratory, consolidating surgery and other specialties such as nephrology and opening a six-bed neonatal intensive care unit. Another suggestion for the long term was to have a free-standing building next to the Foothills Hospital and the Medical School, with physical and program links to the Foothills Hospital. An important proviso was that an independent board of trustees should continue to be in control of the Alberta Children's Hospital, even if relocated.

Professional staff from many different disciplines increased in number throughout the 1970s and the 1980s, with nurses remaining the largest single group. Many of these professionals were combined in an administrative group called the "Treatment Division." The composition of this group varied, and this precise title was not always used. However, the group contributes to all hospital activities, including Prosthetics/Orthotics, Recreation/Child Life, Volunteer Services, Speech and Hearing, Physiotherapy, Occupational Therapy, Psychology, Social Services and Orthoptics. A number of other hospital departments have been in this Division at one time or another, including Radiology, Dental Services, EEG and ECG, Laboratory Services and Respiratory Therapy.

Professionals in all of these disciplines work within the in-patient clusters and in DAT areas as team members and also provide individual care appropriate to their profession. The precise management structure is not important, but in the early days of the hospital, each of these divisions had a director, and there was a considerable administrative overlap. More recently, many of the departments were combined in Psychosocial and Rehabilitative Services, and even this arrangement did not last long.

The Recreation/Child Life Department has varied in size, but helps provide for the psychosocial, emotional and developmental needs of children. Communication and diversion are used to assist in creating an environment sensitive to the special needs of families.

The Speech and Hearing Department has been large[7] and, at one time, provided many of these services to children within Calgary. The department works with children, particularly children with disabilities, to help them communicate their ideas, feelings and emotions effectively. Leadership was provided in innovative ways by Caroline Dunsmore until her retirement. The Hearing Department supports the management of children with hearing impairments through diagnostic assessment, hearing fitting and program planning.

The Physiotherapy Department deals with the prevention and alleviation of physical dysfunction using treatment modalities such as heat, massage, manipulation and active or passive movements. This department was pleased to have the hydrotherapy pool which is also used in treatment.

Occupational Therapy provides intervention for disabilities that interfere with the child's development and habilitation and rehabilitation care, focussing on fine motor adaptive skills, personal and social skills and self-care skills.

The Psychology Department works with children and families on psychological factors, including intellectual, neuropsychological, interpersonal

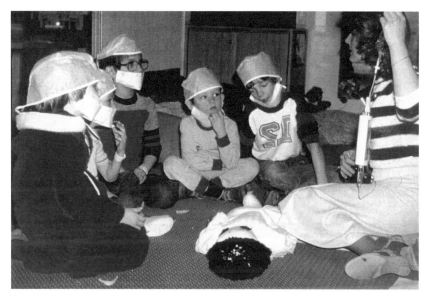

"So ... will this happen to me?"

and emotional functioning and provides treatment through individual group and family therapy. Psychologists, most of whom have doctoral degrees, provide behavior management counselling, social skills training, play therapy and help in the adjustment to disability and chronic illness. This is also an advanced training program to prepare graduates for clinical practice.

The Social Work Department works diligently and co-operatively with health-care professionals to support, strengthen and enhance child and family relationships and also provides family therapy, parent groups, crisis intervention and many other individualized services.

Pastoral care was an issue for many of the parents who were pioneers in forming the Alberta Children's Hospital, and much of the pastoral care was provided by local clergy. The first Chaplain appointed was Reverend Steve Overall, then Reverend Brian Woodrow. The Chaplains were responsible for many services, including the development of an ethics support service and encouraging the development of a small chapel for reflection within the hospital. There is no longer an "ACH Chaplain," but support is provided by the CRHA Department of Pastoral Care. Students within that program are assigned to the ACH site and work with staff and community clergy to provide appropriate care for families.

Photography is an important clinical service which documents congenital anomalies, injuries and illnesses and can record the child's progression as he/she grows and develops. This service, under Carol Petersen, is now much broader and provides a full range of audio-visual services, including videos and advanced slide-making. Audio-visual services are as vital to the educational role of the hospital as they are to clinical services. To support this, the CRHA has agreed to continue a modified service at the ACH site.

One program that uses professionals from many different divisions is the Child Abuse Program. The public recognition of child abuse is recent although the program itself is not. It started in May 1973 but was physically located on the ACH site in May 1982. The program at the Alberta Children's Hospital is active in consultation and assessment in both crisis and long-term treatment, although legal authority for ensuring child protection lies with Provincial Child Welfare Services. The Alberta Children's Hospital program is a leader in research in such areas as aggression management for abusive parents and treatment for sexually abused children and in providing education on child abuse to professional groups. There have been more than a thousand educational presentations over the last twenty years. The many different professionals working closely together include psychologists, social workers, nurses, physicians (paediatricians and child psychiatrists) and also volunteers, who fill an important role. In 1977, Dr. Jack Brummitt, after a time as Acting Director of the DAT Centre, became Director of Child Abuse until 1988, when he was followed by Pat Dougan. When Pat left, Keith Donaghy took over as Manager. The largest number of referrals in any one year was 1,001 in 1992, but this number will probably be exceeded in the year 1996-97.

Orthopaedic surgery was the major activity in the hospital until the 1960s and remains important, representing 11.5 percent of admissions and 10.3 percent of DAT Centre cases. The orthopaedic surgeons have been very supportive of all the changes during the transition from an orthopaedic hospital to a general paediatric hospital. The early orthopaedic surgeons, such as Dr. Deane and Dr. Townsend, played a major role, and their successors have contributed to the major re-development of the hospital. The newer generation of orthopaedic surgeons in the hospital have advanced training in paediatric orthopaedic surgery and confine their practice to the care of children. The present Director of the Division of Paediatric Surgery is an orthopaedic surgeon (Dr. Jim Harder).

The first general paediatric surgeon in Calgary was Dr. Geoff Seagram, who came in 1972. His skills and expertise rapidly became widely recognized, and he had an immediate impact. For extensive periods, he has been the only paediatric surgeon in Calgary, and therefore his skills were particularly needed if there was a neonatal emergency. Dr. Seagram is also a ski enthusiast, and if there happened to be an emergency on weekends, a message would go to the ski hill and Dr. Seagram would return to Calgary. Other general surgeons have included Dr. Steven Rubin (1979 to 1985) and more recently Dr. Andrew Wong and Dr. Robin Eccles.

Neurosurgery has also had prominence in Calgary, and neurosurgeons have contributed to the care of children in the DAT Centre, e.g., spina

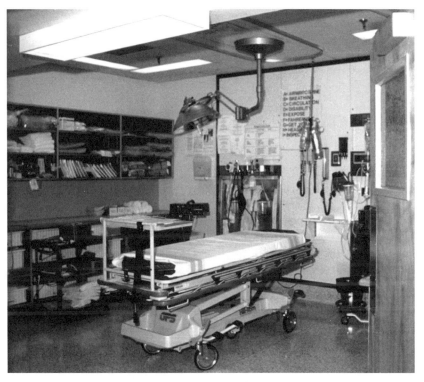

Ready for an emergency.

bifida, as well as being available for major trauma and to treat children with brain cancer. Dr. Terry Myles has been on staff for many years and served as Chief of Staff in the 1980s and early 1990s.

Now there are many other surgical specialists in the Department of Surgery, all of whom contribute to the care of children and include otolaryngologists, ophthalmologists, plastic surgeons and urological surgeons.

Surgery cannot be done without anaesthesia, and the high calibre of work in this area at the Alberta Children's Hospital is a tribute to the many paediatric anaesthetists. When the hospital first opened, such services were provided by anaesthetists who looked after adults and children, but following the appointment of Dr. Gerry Goresky in 1982, the number of full-time paediatric anaesthetists has increased. They have introduced many new techniques and have developed an extensive pain service mainly to deal with the post-operative period, but also for children requiring palliative care. Some of the techniques are effective, but may be difficult to understand outside the setting of a children's hospital. One anaesthetist always tells stories to the children as anaesthesia is being induced. Bubble-gum flavor is commonly used in the anaesthesia mask, making it a tasty experience for children.

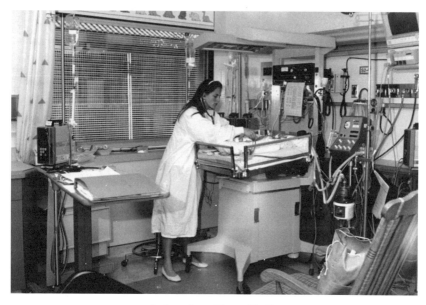

Intensive Care Unit.

The Intensive Care Unit contributes to many parts of the hospital, including children with the most severe illness and patient care after surgery. Directors have been Dr. D.M. Cooper, Dr. I. Mitchell, Dr. Robin Cox and (Acting Director) Dr. Ruth Connors. Multidisciplinary care is provided in the Intensive Care Unit, with strong collaboration from nurses and other professionals, as in other parts of the hospital. There are two major parts in the present Intensive Care Unit, the larger part, the Paediatric Intensive Care Unit, for children beyond the neonatal period, and the small six-bed Neonatal Intensive Care Unit for neonates, particularly those requiring surgery.

The Emergency Department has also undergone many changes and developments over the years. The nurses initially transferred from Foothills Hospital, and some of those nurses continue to work at ACH. The physicians worked at both the Foothills Hospital and the Alberta Children's Hospital and were led by Dr. Greg Powell. Dr. Donald Clogg became the first Paediatric Head of the Emergency Department in 1983, and following his recruitment, many young paediatricians sought to work in this department. The emergency physicians in the department all have expertise and a strong interest in paediatric care. The present Director, Dr. Cheri Nijssen-Jordan, provides a paediatric focus but maintains good relationships with adult trauma services, including the emergency physicians at Foothills Hospital who provide some services.

Oncology has been provided in Calgary and southern Alberta with the original vision of Dr. R. Truscott. Shortly before the Alberta Children's

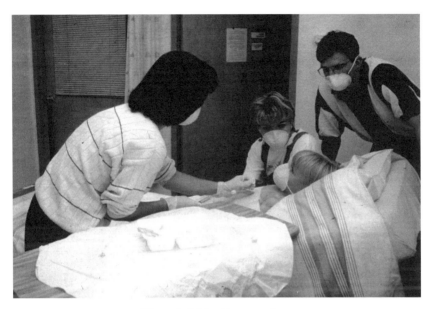

The child in the centre.

Hospital opened, Dr. Ted Zipf was recruited as Director of Oncology, providing care at the Alberta Children's Hospital (from 1982 onwards) and for out-patients at the Tom Baker Cancer Centre. The split service was united with the opening of the Oncology Outpatient Clinic in 1990, under the directorship of Dr. Ron Grant. The current Director is Dr. Max Coppes. The treatment offered in Oncology is now advanced, requiring a high level of supervision, and the newly renovated out-patient clinic is carefully designed so that there is the right physical ambiance for the high level of supervision required. A new development in oncology is bone marrow transplant, developed under the leadership of Dr. Tom Bowen and Dr. Jim Russell and continued as an integral part of the Oncology Program after Dr. Bowen's departure. Bone marrow transplants are used in cancer treatment for children no longer responsive to chemotherapy and in a number of genetic and immunological diseases. The Oncology Service has integrated medical and nursing care and a high level of psychosocial support. Its success depends on almost all services of the Child Health Centre, and its association with The University of Calgary and the Tom Baker Cancer Centre allows research to be pursued. There is a parent group, the Candlelighters, in the Oncology Service, as there is in many other services who work closely with health-care professionals.

The present-day Genetic Service continues to be a model of community and preventive service, with roots in the 1970s. Genetic services were reviewed by a number of committees, the first set up by Dr. W.A.

Cochrane (who became Deputy Minister of Health after a term as Dean of Medicine at The University of Calgary) in 1974. The committee, chaired by Dr. John Read, recommended that there be a provincial genetic service providing both clinical and laboratory services, with specific designated funding.[8] Services were to be provided not only in Calgary and Edmonton, but also in public health clinics throughout the province. There was to be laboratory back-up and a provincial metabolic screening program. The funds were provided directly by the government, separate from hospital grants, but administered by the Alberta Children's Hospital and the University of Alberta Hospital. The department in Calgary has been led by Dr. Brian Lowry from the beginning, and in addition to the clinicians, the original group included Dr. C.C. (Jim) Lin (Cytogenetics,) and Dr. F. Snyder (Biochemical Genetics). Others recruited contribute to the genetics, cytogenetics and research laboratories. Many have achieved prominence for their research achievements including Dr. Leigh Field and Dr. Renee Martin. The Department of Genetics maintains a Vital Statistics registry for all children with congenital anomalies, and this information is used in monitoring disease. The importance of genetics was recognized by The University of Calgary which created a Genetics Department distinct from Paediatrics in 1993.

Many medical services and divisions developed throughout the 1980s and 1990s. For example, Dr. R.H.A. Haslam, in addition to being Department Head, was a well-known paediatric neurologist. He was particularly noted as a gifted teacher. Dr. Harvey Sarnat then Dr. Hussam Darwish have followed as Division Directors. In Gastroenterology, Dr. Grant Gall, followed by Dr. Brent Scott, were Division Directors, and both combine clinical care with laboratory research. Dr. R. McArthur, the first endocrinologist, has been succeeded as Division Director by Dr. D. Stephure. Respirology was originally combined with ICU care (Dr. D.M. Cooper) but now is a separate division (Dr. I. Mitchell, Director) and provides a wide range of services, supported by committed nurses and respiratory therapists. Developmental Paediatrics has been led by Dr. J. Fagan and Dr. M. Clarke, but many general paediatricians work in the division. Nephrology services were limited until Dr. Raymond Donckerwolcke, who was already internationally known, was recruited recently. Infectious Disease services were provided by Dr. Ken Buchan originally, but Dr. Taj Jadavji was the first full-time paediatric infectious disease physician, and he has been joined by well-trained colleagues. General paediatric services continue at a high level, mainly provided by community paediatricians.

Cardiac diseases cause great anxiety to professionals and parents. This division was headed by Dr. R. Somerville and now by Dr. Joyce Harder. The Cardiac Division has been a pioneer in using non-invasive and safe tests in children, and, in particular, ultrasound has been very successful in reducing the number of invasive and thus risky procedures. Cardiology

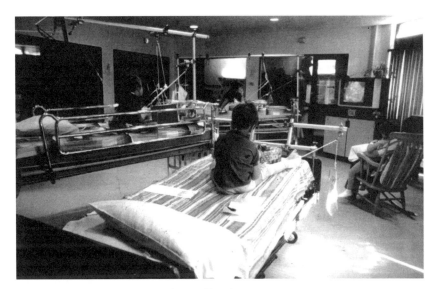

In-patient area.

is provided as a provincial service, and cardiologists in Calgary work closely with cardiologists and cardiac surgeons in Edmonton. With the opening of the cardiac catheterization laboratory (Special Procedures Room), most investigations can be completed at the Alberta Children's Hospital, with a transfer to the University of Alberta Hospital for those children who require surgery.

Not all medical services are described, and choosing to describe a few individuals and a few of the medical divisions does not mean these are the only important ones or that care is compartmentalized. Nothing could be further from the truth. Not only do physicians from different divisions work closely together, all depend on nursing colleagues, professionals from many disciplines and support staff.

The "Diagnostic Imaging Department" is the new name for the X-ray Department, and the title indicates that there are many different ways of obtaining pictures of the inside of children's bodies. While there had been a small department on the 17th Avenue site for many years, the department was updated when Dr. Richard Wesenberg was appointed Director in 1979. He amassed appropriate equipment and was particularly interested in low-dose radiation. His prestige was enough to recruit excellent colleagues, and the department remained under good and capable hands when Dr. Wesenberg left as he was wanted in quite a few other places. The present Director is Dr. Graham Boag. Dr. Dagmar Mueller was Acting Director for some time between the two directors and remains a member of the department. One of the obvious deficiencies of the department in the early years was a lack of a CT scanner, but one was eventually installed in 1987. One form of imaging not obtained for ACH is an MRI scanner, which uses magnetic fields to give detailed pictures of the body without radiation and is thus particularly suitable for children. However, it was decided that this equipment should be in adult hospitals only, and children are transferred for the test.

Laboratories is a name which means different things to different people. The public often think of them as the place where the specimen is collected, but for the professionals, laboratories are where specimens are analyzed. Until recently, there were a full range of laboratories at the Alberta Children's Hospital, dealing with all aspects of patient care. Recent cutbacks have meant that many of the laboratories are off-site, with only a few specific laboratories at the Alberta Children's Hospital. Information from laboratories is needed quickly when children are acutely ill. One service, for example, involves examining surgical specimens while the patient is still anaesthetized and using the results to guide the extent of surgery. The pathologists are Dr. Cynthia Trevenen and Dr. Alfredo Pinto, and Dr. Dierdre Church is microbiologist.

Psychiatry is a medical service, part of the Mental Health Service, and relates closely to Psychology, Social Work, Family Therapy, Child Abuse and so on. Dr. Tim Yates was one of the early heads of Psychiatry, succeeded by Dr. Phil Barker, although the position is presently vacant. The Child Psychiatry Department deals with issues of rehabilitation of children with mental illness and generally does not see children above the age of twelve. Much of the practice of child psychiatry is as out-patients, including a day program using facilities in the Dr. Gordon Townsend School, but there is a small in-patient component. This was initially in H Cluster, but is now in the purpose-built W Cluster near the Dr. Gordon Townsend School.

Modern paediatric services use drugs, which must be correctly chosen and delivered in precise doses because children, partly because of their size, may be affected by even small errors. Up to 1958, the pharmacy service was provided by calling an outside pharmacist to the hospital. At this time, the medication itself was measured out by the matron in the basement and delivered to the wards. Later, at the opening of the new extension in 1981, a Director of Pharmacy (Elaine McKenzie) was appointed, and there was a change in the practice of dispensing drugs when unit dose treatment was introduced. This was a sharp change with tradition, in which stocks of drugs were kept on the ward and nurses measured out the dose and gave it to the child. Now, under the unit dose system, specific doses are made for a child in the pharmacy, sealed and sent labelled to the ward. Donna Pipa was appointed Director in 1984, and since then pharmacists have become closely involved as part of the team caring for all in-patients, particularly in the Intensive Care Unit. Oncology not only requires a pharmacist dedicated to the in-patient and out-patient areas, but has its own out-patient pharmacy. All the pharmacists are fully involved in providing continuing education for the staff of the hospital.

Rapid access to knowledge is essential if a high level of care is given, and thus libraries have a major role in all hospitals. Librarians use computerized literature searches to retrieve the latest information required for the care of children and can provide this for staff. At ACH, Barbara Hatt provided those services and others such as helping staff (at all levels) with preparation for presentations and helping parents find more information on their child's condition. The librarian helped in obtaining some information required for this history. It has been decided that ACH does not need a librarian for its library.

The administration of the hospital remains important, but there have been many changes. Leadership in the new hospital of 1981-82 was provided by Robert Innes (appointed in 1972) whose vision was responsible for the present-day service and who worked extensively with all groups of staff in developing an appropriate model of care. On the other hand, he had continuing problems with medical staff dating back as far as 1975, when the staff felt they had little input in planning. In 1987, a number of physicians complained publicly about conditions at the hospital. There were also increasing financial pressures in the late 1980s, and Robert Innes resigned[9] in 1989 and was replaced by Jim Saunders, who was given the title of President. Jim Saunders was an administrator within the Calgary hospital system with general experience, rather than specific experience in paediatric health care. He concentrated on improving both his own knowledge of paediatrics and the financial management of the hospital. He was able to see the financial cutbacks through with minimal disturbance, certainly a tribute to his leadership skills. For a short period, there was a Vice-President, Medical Services, an appointment created following the recommendations of the Haggerty Report. The administration of the Alberta Children's Hospital changed dramatically after the development of the CRHA. Most of the senior administrators left. Nora Greenley, who had been Vice-President, Patient Care Services, became Senior Operating Officer for the Child Health Program (and for other programs).

The Alberta Children's Hospital Foundation was formed in 1972 after the provincial government took over ACH, and, for the next ten years, its major role was trustee for funding paid for the hospital and bequests to the hospital. Total bequests varied from a high of $354,813 in 1983[10] to a low of $37,621 in 1976.[11] Overall in the period 1973 to 1984, $1,301,389 was donated. Between bequest and investment income, the ACHF was able to assist the development of the Alberta Children's Hospital in the 1970s and to fund additional services in the 1980s. It contributed to the major expansion in 1982. Income available to the Foundation in 1973 was $465,202 and first broke the $1 million mark in 1982 ($1,071,962).

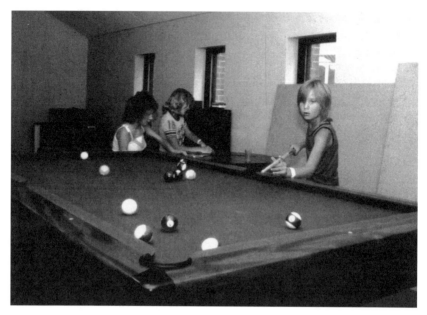

Recreation for in-patients.

At that time, the main expenditures were Research Centre costs, research grants and research and travelling fellowships. The ACHF sought a greater role, and one of its initiatives was the Chair in Paediatric Research. Julius Lister was appointed Executive Director and explored a number of new initiatives, including the Miracle Network Telethon. There were many discussions over 1984-85 involving many players and all of the local television stations. CFAC became a major sponsor led by Ed Whalen. The first telethon in 1985 stimulated donations of $57,000, and the telethon, under the leadership of John Huggett (appointed November 14, 1985), became the centrepiece of a fundraising effort. Half a million dollars were raised in 1986, and now the telethon receives over $1 million in donations annually. There are may different fundraising activities within the ACH Foundation, including the Kinsmen Home Lotto, golf tournament (CHAS), Stampede Marathon Race, Festival of Lights and Wear your Bear Campaign. Now the ACH Foundation works within the CRHA, which seems to have accepted the need for a specific fundraising organization for sick children.

There will be further developments in service delivery as Calgary itself and paediatrics change. The Alberta Children's Hospital will provide services by the year 2000 to about 230,000 children under nineteen years of age in Calgary and its immediate region and to about 400,000 in the whole of southern Alberta. There will be substantial numbers in every age group, with slightly more adolescents and slightly fewer infants than

Emily

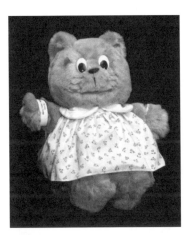

B y the 1970s, it was accepted that going to a hospital caused children anxiety and that sometimes spending time there could be as traumatic as the actual injury or illness. If children knew what was happening to them, then the hospital and illness could be less threatening, but it was not clear exactly how to provide that information to children. Janice Robertson (Director of Child Life) discussed this topic with Lorna Fraser, and the idea of a kitten was developed. The kitten was a good listener, cuddly and trustworthy, reflecting the warm, devoted and friendly atmosphere of the Alberta Children's Hospital. Children named her after a contest throughout the hospital; "Emily" was by far the favorite name. The first coloring book, "Emily Goes to the Hospital," was produced in 1976 to introduce children to the hospital and medical instruments. Following the coloring book, there was a puppet show in 1977, as a pre-operative and assessment program. The star was, of course, Emily, and a child was followed from admission to the hospital right through to discharge. This show continued for many, many years before being replaced.

A teddy-bear program was later started to introduce "well" children to the hospital, and children from kindergartens around Calgary come for a familiarization tour.

Emily is now a familiar figure in the daily life of the Alberta Children's Hospital, with Emily's Window, Emily's Backyard, Emily's Toybox – where donations can be dropped off – and Emily's Hotline, where advice is given on emergencies in children. Of course, Emily was present when the new Child Health Centre opened in 1981 as a stuffed toy with a change of clothes to reflect all of the seasons. In 1988, she was sold as a fundraiser in collaboration with the Bank of Montreal. She still symbolizes all the hospital represents.

Emily may be superseded by new images, but will not be replaced in the hearts of many generations of children.

before. Immigrants will remain a vital force in the life of Calgary, and quite a few will speak little English. Not only is an increase in single-parent families expected, but there will also be more low-income families with one or more children. However, the present high level of out-patient care activity (771,000 visits in 1995-96) will continue. The major conditions treated may change. In 1995-96, these were tonsillitis, asthma, bronchiolitis, gastroenteritis, pneumonia, croup, appendicitis, orthopaedic conditions and cancer. Whatever the patient's medical condition or personal background, ACH will meet the need. Staff will continue to strive to improve and develop services, always with a commitment to the needs of the whole child.❖

References

1. Health Records, Alberta Children's Hospital, 1997.
2. Human Resources, Alberta Children's Hospital, 1997.
3. Bonham, A. *Review of Medical Services*, Alberta Children's Hospital 1983.
4. Finance Department, Alberta Children's Hospital, 1996.
5. *The Calgary Herald*, December 3, 1996, p. A11.
6. Resources Management Consultants (Alberta) Ltd. Report of the Subcommittee of the Calgary Area Hospital Advisory Council (CAHAC) to the CAHAC and Alberta Children's Hospital Board, May 7, 1987.
7. *The Calgary Herald*, May 19, 1985, p. D5.
8. Read Report on Hereditary Diseases to the Minister of Health, March, 1976.
9. Innes, R. Letter to staff, March 21, 1989.
10. *Annual Report*. Alberta Children's Hospital Foundation , 1983.
11. *Annual Report*. Alberta Children's Hospital Foundation, 1976.
12. *Annual Report*. Alberta Children's Hospital Foundation, 1982.

Changes to the New Building

The hospital in 1997, both from the outside and the inside, looks similar to 1982. There have been, however, many alterations and one large extension which moved the front of the hospital closer to Richmond Road. This extension came about after the Haggerty Committee recommendations (p. 175) were accepted by the government. Additions immediately outside the hospital, such as the swimming pool and helipad, and several blocks away (Ronald McDonald House) are all essential parts of the hospital service, added in the 1980s.

The addition at the front and, in particular, the new oncology clinic were significant in the life of the hospital. Many patients, over many years, recognized that the organization for the care of cancer patients could be better, although the care itself was of the highest possible standard. These children, and their families, had in-patient care for cancer at the Alberta Children's Hospital, but, as out-patients, went to the Tom Baker Cancer Centre. Now these children can attend the new out-patient clinic immediately inside the main entrance. The location was chosen to minimize the chance of exposure to infectious disease, because children with cancer, particularly if they are in treatment, are highly vulnerable to

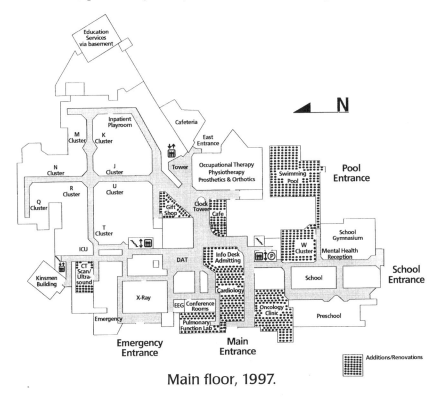

Main floor, 1997.

infection, and even childhood illnesses such as chicken pox can have major complications. The inside of the oncology clinic is bright and airy. On one side are rooms for physician examination and, beyond these rooms, a comfortable lounge. On the other side is space for children to have day treatment. There are complete facilities to make the stay as comfortable as possible and to carry out procedures safely. The new clinic is some distance from the ward inside the hospital where children are admitted, but staff are shared between the two units, and the children know all of the staff well.

The cardiology and pulmonary function laboratories are also off the new entrance hall, opposite the oncology clinic. The cardiology area has clinic rooms and a room for echocardiography (ultrasound), which is important in the investigation of suspected heart disease. The technician or cardiologist uses a small probe placed against the skin to see, with the greatest of detail, the activity of the heart, and how it is constructed. The room in which this test is done has a VCR with appropriate movies and cartoon videos. Some children may require more extensive investigations in the Special Procedures Room, but the echocardiogram can help limit those investigations. A treadmill is nearby for exercise-testing of children with heart or lung disease. Generally the staff are happy that the children, rather than they themselves, run on the treadmill! In the pulmonary function laboratory, children are exhorted by the technician to breathe harder, harder and harder. Immediately beyond this noisy area is the sleep laboratory, where children with sleep disorders can be studied. This room is, of course, soundproof.

In the main hallway, the entrance to the Scarborough Clinic can be seen. There has been a public health clinic for immunization and routine examination of children in the neighborhood of the hospital, but now it is actually within the hospital. This helps the liaison with hospital staff. Immediately beyond the Scarborough Clinic is the security office and information desk, where staff give directions to help visitors find their way through the maze of the hospital. At the end of the hallway is a bright stained-glass window, dedicated to all the patients of the hospital. In the same area, next to the elevators, are the offices of the Alberta Children's Hospital Foundation and the entrance to the school.

One of the many changes to the school over the years, has been the relocation of the Mental Health In-patient Cluster to W Cluster, which took place in 1990. Here, children with emotional, behavioral and mental problems are admitted to purpose-designed facilities. This cluster operates five days a week, and the children are glad to go home for the weekend. The atmosphere in the ward is informal, and in addition to psychiatric treatment and assessment, there is a close connection with the school to continue education and also with

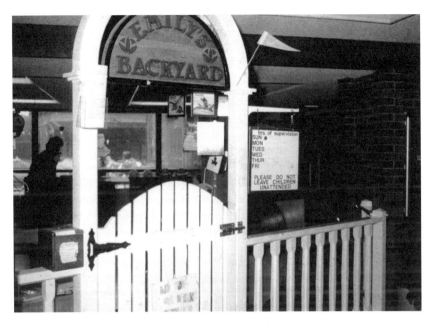

Emily's backyard.

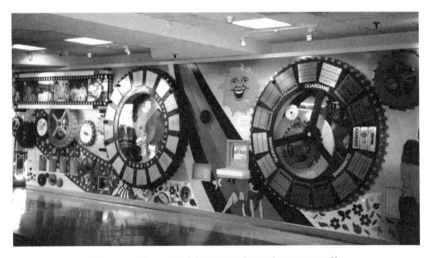

Innovative and interactive donor wall.

services such as occupational therapy. There is accommodation for a day treatment program, an aspect that could be expanded further.

Beyond the main information desk in the direction of the DAT Centre, there is now a donor wall. Most hospitals honor those who have given a bequest or donated money by inscribing their name on a plaque whose size and prominence is related to the amount of money given. In previous

Alberta Children's Hospital buildings, these plaques were placed on the end of a crib or on the door of a ward. Now, donors are still honored, but the area is full of action toys that children can play with and move. This is surely one of the most innovative donor walls anywhere, appropriate for a children's hospital. It is often difficult to try and take a child away from it as parents try to go to one of the many hospital departments. Immediately opposite the donor wall is Emily's Backyard, a play area for children run by volunteers who look after siblings while parents are busy with a child in the hospital, another area where children really want to stay!

The DAT area is beyond the donor wall and Emily's Backyard. One of the eyecatchers is the vinyl flooring, which has recently been laid extensively throughout the hospital, not just in the DAT Centre; several hundreds of thousands of dollars have been spent replacing carpet. The patient service area is in the middle of the DAT Centre, and immediately beyond that area is the fish tank. A previous fish tank had leaks, and it was thought to be too expensive to replace. Parents put pressure on the Alberta Children's Hospital Foundation to pay for a new fish tank, and ultimately the Foundation was pleased to do so. Parents had pointed out that this was one of the few living things in the area that children could look at while they waited for their appointment. Certainly, the fish tank and all the other amenities and toys in the DAT area mean that children are comfortable and happy to attend the hospital and tend to be cooperative in their appointments with professionals. This is so important that in a recent meeting to discuss changes to a clinic area, space in which children would draw with crayons had the same priority as the rooms for medical examination or nursing assessment.

Many of the DAT clinics have been remodelled, and further remodelling will occur as the various services change in response to changes in practice and new technology. For example, investigations are now more likely to be completed as an out-patient, but sedation is often required. Thus special arrangements are required for the supervision of the child until full recovery. Another change is a considerable increase in the amount of patient and parent education provided. While this has always been a priority, it now requires much more dedicated space.

The Diagnostic Imaging Department is beyond the DAT area, and one of the early and major developments was the acquisition of the CT scanner. Medical staff had pressed for this for some years, and once it was acquired, children with major trauma did not need to be transported, while unstable, to another facility.

The Emergency Department has been renovated on a number of occasions. The observation ward opened in 1987[1] for children with illnesses such as severe diarrhea leading to dehydration, croup or asthma, who may be admitted for a few hours for intensive treatment. Improvement usually allows discharge home, although some children may be admitted to hospital from the observation ward. Most parents do not mind spending a few hours with their child, knowing that they may eventually be able to go home. The Emergency Department, the designated trauma centre for children, has full facilities for dealing with major injuries. However, further alterations and improvements are planned to ensure that treatment remains optimal.

The chapel is beyond the Emergency Department and immediately adjacent to the in-patient area. It was formerly a lounge for paediatric residents, but the alteration came about due to considerable pressure to offer more provision for the spiritual dimension of care offered. The chapel was developed as a place of quiet reflection for parents or staff of any, or no, religious domination.

In the in-patient area, only a few of the many changes are obvious. The Paediatric Intensive Care Unit (PICU) has been changed considerably. Originally there were two areas, an acute area with seven beds and a progressive area with eight beds. In 1990-91, the acute area was expanded to nine beds, and a six-bed Neonatal Intensive Care Unit (NICU) was added. Infants with major congenital anomalies requiring surgery are admitted to this unit for pre- and post-operative care. An area planned as a progressive/stepdown unit for both PICU and NICU is immediately beyond the NICU, but is presently used for day surgery.

Crossroads is still the physical centre of the in-patient area, but there is no longer a desk or a receptionist to deal with clerical functions for all the clusters. The units now have their own clerical staff, and Crossroads only has a phone for use of visitors and staff who require help or direction. Many of the clusters have had major internal modifications. Twelve-bed clusters have been combined to form twenty-three- and twenty-four-bed clusters. The first twinning of clusters took place in 1992, when P and N were twinned into one cluster called N. This alteration was intended to provide more opportunities for nurses to develop higher skill levels, to reduce management costs and to provide a designated area where professionals could complete charts and discuss patients without interfering with the space for children. Twinning has been successful in achieving most of these objectives, although there is little doubt that there was a loss of the intimate atmosphere of the smaller clusters. Further twinnings occurred in 1993 and 1995.

The oncology ward has had major alterations on more than one occasion and has been alternately located in M Cluster and Q Cluster. The alterations were to meet specialized patient care needs. There are also more patients attending this area, partly due to the success of treatment leading to longer survival and partly because of the location of the provincial bone marrow transplant program for children at the Alberta Children's Hospital. In this area, special attention is paid to measures to reduce the risk of infection to these vulnerable children, so, for example,

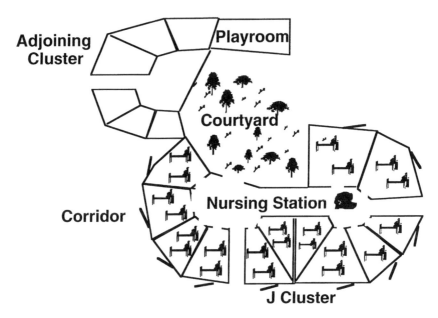

Plan of twinned clusters.

there is extra air filtration. The rooms are mainly single rooms, and as children have to spend a long time in one room, the rooms themselves are as comfortable and welcoming as possible. There is a lounge for parents and visitors to maintain the atmosphere of home-like care, which continues to be part of the hospital's philosophy.

On a circular tour from the in-patient area and Crossroads back toward the Child Space, we pass the new play area, where there are a number of attractive toys and a large train mural. On the edge of the Child Space is the Prosthetic/Orthotic Department, one of the departments present almost since the opening of the hospital, originally as the brace-maker shop but now with a wide variety of functions. Also in the same area is the store, Emily's Window, where volunteers sell toys and books and other useful items.

In the Child Space is the Main Street Cafe, a recent addition, where many staff and parents go for informal coffee breaks and snacks. Immediately beyond the Main Street Cafe is an outside paved area, which, given Calgary's weather, is used mainly in the short summer months, but is a welcome area in the middle of a busy day where staff can have lunch. Parents and children also enjoy the opportunity to go outside with a minimum of fuss.

There have been changes in the basement. The pharmacy, for example, has enlarged considerably to deal with the demands of all the new services. There are now special arrangements for preparing parenteral

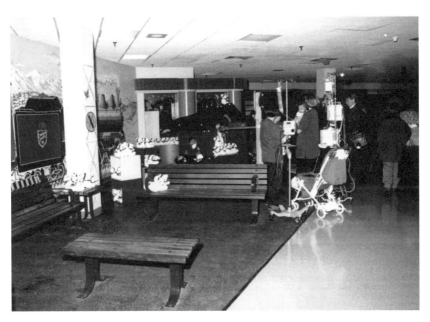

"Let's get the train out of here!"

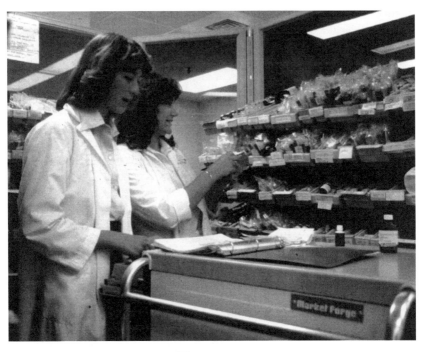

Pharmacy.

feeding (food which goes into the vein of the child) as this can easily be contaminated by infection. The pharmacy also has a large information section, again as part of the enhanced service to make sure that children get the best possible care. The out-patient section of the pharmacy is near the information desk on the first floor.

One exciting development in the basement is the Hubert Richardson Wing. This was built with a bequest by Hubert Richardson, a farmer in southern Alberta with no children of his own, who felt that the money he had amassed over the years could best be given to children. This wing was opened on April 14, 1988,[2] and has first-class facilities for genetic research. The opening ceremony was conducted by Dave Russell, who at that time was Minister of Advanced Education, but had been the Minister of Hospitals at the time of the expansion in 1982.

One area of the hospital with an uncertain future is the laboratory. Much of the testing is now being done off site in the newly created Calgary Laboratory Service, although some laboratory testing continues on the ACH site. Children may briefly attend the new phlebotomy lab to have blood taken, though the sample may be tested at ACH or elsewhere.

On the second floor, there are a number of alterations, some of which are obvious such as the dental suite, and some are less obvious. As part of the extension at the front opened in 1990, there were new meeting rooms and offices for Psychology and Social Work. In part of the shell space created in 1979-80 with the money from the federal sales tax rebate, there are physicians' offices and, more importantly, accommodation for the paediatric residents. The residents perform an essential function in any hospital, all being qualified physicians, undergoing advanced training in paediatrics or other specialties and present in the hospital twenty-four hours a day. For many years after the hospital opened in 1982, accommodation for residents was little more than a converted closet, and purpose-built sleep rooms and lounges are needed to support a vital service.

On the second floor is also the Audiology Department which was relocated to allow the Ophthalmology and Orthoptic Clinics to combine and is now located next to Speech Therapy.

The Operating Rooms have expanded to include an additional Operating Room added recently, with state-of-the-art equipment. The most recent opening at the Alberta Children's Hospital (November 1996) was the Special Procedures Room. Public and professionals felt it was needed to make the investigation of vulnerable children safer. Here we find state-of-the-art equipment to assess cardiac function and anatomy, requiring catheters to be inserted into the infant's heart and dye injected. The same equipment is used to study blood vessels (angiograph) in, for example, major trauma. This is clearly a high-risk procedure and should be located inside the operating room suite, where facilities are available should further help be needed, and immediately above the PICU.

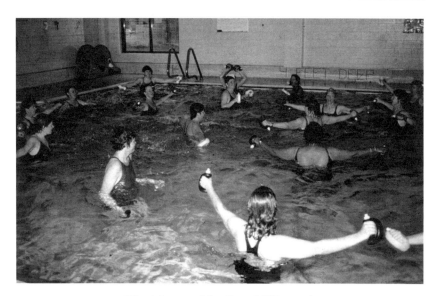

Working out in the ACH pool.

The swimming pool on the southeast side of the hospital opened in June 1984,[3] but was proposed as long ago as 1941.[4] At that time, the importance of aquatherapy was recognized, and a Hubbard tank was installed. Planning for the swimming pool started in 1977,[5] and a detailed proposal was submitted jointly by the Rotary Club and CHAS on February 7, 1979. Though it remains popular, the swimming pool is now used by the public more than by hospital patients. The water tends to be slightly warmer than in most public pools. However, many feel that it does not belong on hospital property and should not be subsidized in any way by hospital money.

A hostel for parents was one of the aims of the planners in the 1970s, but was not provided until Ronald McDonald House opened at 1921 – 28th Street SW in March 1985. The government donated the land on which the house was built, and major donors included the Lions Club, the Junior League of Calgary and, of course, McDonald's Restaurants. This home away from home is to be used by families from southern Alberta or southeastern British Columbia whose child is undergoing treatment or diagnostic examinations.[6]

The helipad is at the front of the hospital near Crowchild Trail. When a helicopter is not there, only a flat concrete pad and a windsock above the Emergency Department give a clue to its function. The helipad itself was developed after extensive discussions with the local community, which was concerned that it would be over-used and there would be a considerable increase in noise. The hospital staff were sensitive to this concern and continue to scrutinize transport closely to ensure that it is used when

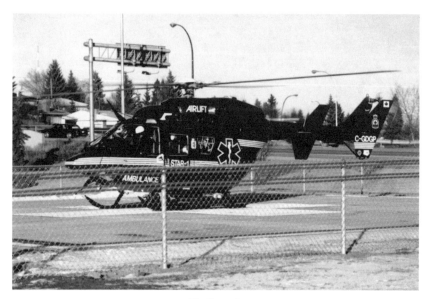

Helipad.

appropriate to save life or limb. When transport is required, hospital security and police combine efforts to stop traffic. The helicopter lands,
and quickly the staff who accompanied the child climb out, place the
child on a trolley and cross the road without delay to take the child to the
Emergency Department, where assessment continues in the major trauma
area or children go directly to PICU. The helicopter takes off, and traffic
flow resumes. Before the helipad was in place, helicopters landed at the
naval base at Tecumseh which is across Crowchild Trail, so there was
some extra handling of the child required to travel by ambulance to the
Alberta Children's Hospital. The transport of sick and injured children is
an important part of the PICU. Children with severe illnesses who require
intensive care may be seen first at their local hospital anywhere in southern Alberta or southeastern British Columbia. When help is required,
physicians call the staff at the PICU at ACH, who may go and pick up the
child. This service is used between seventy and one hundred times per
year, using ground ambulance, helicopter or fixed wing aircraft as necessary.[7] There are about fifty landings at the helipad per year, using the
helicopter of the Shock Trauma Air Rescue Service (STARS).

There is little doubt that, over the years, the Alberta Children's Hospital will require more alterations and additions to ensure that the highest
standard of care is provided to children in southern Alberta and that the
building changes to accommodate paediatric practice changes.❖

References

1. Alberta Children's Hospital Role Statement, June 30, 1991.
2. Ibid.
3. Ibid.
4. *Minutes*. Executive Committee, Alberta Division, Canadian Red Cross Society, November 15, 1941, p. 3.
5. *Minutes*. Alberta Children's Hospital Foundation Board, December 12, 1978.
6. *The Mirror*, July 16 and October 22, 1984, and *The Calgary Herald*, March 21, 1984.
7. Alberta Children's Hospital Transport Committee, July 15, 1997.

Further reading

Soltan, H.C., ed. *Medical Genetics in Canada: Essay on the Early History*. University of Western Ontario, London, Ontario, 1992.

The History of Pharmacy in Alberta: The First One Hundred Years. The Alberta Pharmaceutical Association, Edmonton, Alberta, 1993.

Alberta Children's Hospital Fights for its Life –1994

"The Alberta Children's Hospital will remain at its present site and continue to offer current programs." This announcement by Health Minister Shirley McLelland was a successful end to a public campaign to prevent the closure of the hospital.[1] Parents and the public were supportive of the hospital, and paediatric health-care providers were almost unanimous in their support. The opposition had been subtle and behind the scenes, mainly by a minority of government bureaucrats and Board members and administrators of the other hospitals in Calgary, none of whom were likely to call publicly for the closure of the Alberta Children's Hospital. A detailed financial analysis confirmed the high cost of converting premises at the Foothills Hospital site suitable for children. In the end, the close link between the Alberta Children's Hospital and the people of Calgary and southern Alberta was the major factor in the decision not to close the Alberta Children's Hospital.

The pressure to close the Alberta Children's Hospital was not simply related to funding cutbacks. For example, there was interest in health-care reform throughout Canada. The major groups involved, such as consumers, physicians, nurses and other health-care professionals, politicians, bureaucrats and academics, often had contradictory views, and there were significant disagreements even within groups. Some of the concerns were: lack of attention to prevention; lack of resources for community care; too great a focus on disease and high technology, thus too much spending on high-technology institutions; and the continuing dominant role of physicians in the system overall and in their relationship with other health-care professionals. Canadians generally expressed a high level of satisfaction with "their" health-care system. There were complaints, of course, but they tended to be about specific incidents rather than the system as a whole.

The Alberta Children's Hospital had participated in a province-wide effort to "reform" the health-care system for children. There had been a wide-ranging inquiry involving all the communities of Alberta and the Child Health Centre of Northern Alberta in addition to the Alberta Children's Hospital Child Health Centre. A provincial paediatric plan was developed and presented to government,[2] but was not accepted because the government had its own plans for health-care changes. In Calgary, paediatric caregivers met regularly to discuss common issues, increasing understanding of the problems faced by different institutions. Yet there were strict limits on co-operation because several distinct boards were involved.

General concerns about children's hospitals throughout the western world also affected ACH. These hospitals were regarded as expensive and too specialized, and many political and academic leaders felt that independent children's hospitals should be replaced by a paediatric unit within a large general hospital. In such a hospital, children's services would be a minority and might very well have a low priority. In common with other children's hospitals, the Alberta Children's Hospital has had extensive ambulatory care and outreach services requiring slightly more than half its budget. This approach was so different from the other general hospitals in Calgary that it was not well understood and led to criticism. Now, with present attitudes to health-care reform, such support for out-patient care seemed vindicated.

It cannot be denied however that financial cutbacks were at the root of the threatened closure of the Alberta Children's Hospital. The Progressive Conservative government elected under the leadership of Ralph Klein in 1992 intended to balance the provincial budget by reducing spending.[3] The Progressive Conservative party had been in power since August 30, 1971,[4] and during the Lougheed years (1971–85) revenues had increased enormously in a booming economy, and there had been increases in spending to support major developments intended to lead to improvements in the lives of Albertans. One of these developments was the expansion of the Alberta Children's Hospital, but there were innumerable other examples throughout the province of government spending on roads, schools and hospitals. Some are examples of unwise spending. Rural hospitals built were described as "spectacularly effective as government gifts, but many of them are extremely inefficient as hospitals with legitimate medical merit."[5] In addition to spending for public service, there were many grants and loans to private industry. From 1984/85 onward, there was a decline in oil prices and thus a considerable drop in government revenue. There were some spending reductions, but grants were still made to business interests, and there was an increase in the provincial deficit to $2.7 billion in 1993, which required large interest payments (9.1 percent of all government spending).[6] Three large departments – Health, Education and Social Services – together accounted for 61.5 percent of government spending. The Department of Health had the largest single budget of any government department, representing almost one-third of all spending. Therefore a significant reduction in government spending could not occur without major cuts to the health-care budget. Such cuts were applied almost as soon as the government was elected. Money transferred from the government to each hospital was progressively reduced, and, although the government did not favor one hospital in particular, the cuts were higher in Calgary and Edmonton than in the rural areas. The government stated that there was "more fat in administration" in the cities, but many felt another factor was the strength of government support in rural Alberta.

All of the Calgary hospitals had to respond quickly to the general cut in transfer payments from the government. The Alberta Children's Hospital received $58,887,429 in 1992/93 and $48,420,021 in 1994/95[7], and this reduction of almost twenty percent meant bed closures, a marked reduction in the number of managers, transfer of some charges to parents, restructuring the delivery of care and close scrutiny of the efficiency of the hospital. One example was the closure of one of the twelve-bed inpatient units, T Cluster, in the Alberta Children's Hospital, which produced annual savings of $85,000. This unit specialized in the care of infants with heart and lung disease. Some of these infants were admitted several times, and the parents took comfort in the fact that the staff knew their child well. Parents were frightened that their child's care would be compromised, and their extreme anxiety reached the press. None of the nurses lost their jobs, as they were all offered positions on other units, and the children were well cared for in another cluster. Nevertheless, events such as these led to fear in staff and parents alike and show that budget cuts not only have a financial effect, but reach the hearts of those involved.

All the hospitals in Calgary offered a high level of care to their patients, but there was duplication and competition as a result of the many separate hospital boards. There were other important health-care agencies in Calgary (nursing homes, Calgary Health Services and the Tom Baker Cancer Centre) and many private organizations which played an important role in overall health-care delivery and, in particular, in providing care for patients who might otherwise be in an acute-care hospital. Many hospitals and agencies were interdependent, but, in the end, each organization was likely to follow its own priorities. The magnitude of the cuts, however, made full co-operation essential. Savings could be made by reducing duplication and, where possible, sharing functions and thus minimizing the impact of cutbacks on direct patient care. The hospital boards and chief executives met as a group throughout the period of budget cuts and restructuring. One of their actions was to form a subcommittee of the Vice Presidents of Medicine and Patient Care Service from each hospital to determine priorities and look at ways services could be rationalized. Although these discussions were fruitful, it was recognized that help was needed, and external consultants (Price Waterhouse) were hired to analyse medical services in Calgary and make recommendations.[8] These attempts at co-operation and the hiring of external consultants were all with the full support of the Government of Alberta.

Price Waterhouse was charged with analysing services (and their costs) in Calgary and developing a number of alternatives. They produced five "configurations" of hospitals, with the Foothills, Rockyview and Peter Lougheed hospitals present in all scenarios. The Alberta Children's Hospital was retained in only one. Cost savings were estimated at $91.4 million per year for Option 1 (Foothills Hospital, Rockyview Hospital and Peter Lougheed Centre), and $81.1 million per year for these three and the Alberta Children's Hospital.[9]

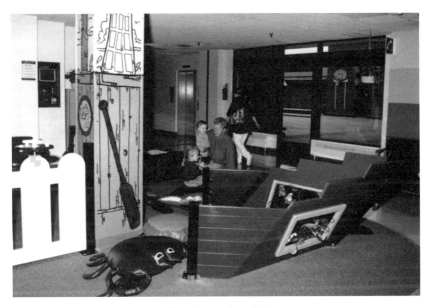

"Let's pretend."

The hospitals made a number of attempts to implement the findings of the Price Waterhouse study but failed to reach agreement. Thus, with the agreement of the government, yet another external group was hired. This group was chaired by Lou Hyndman, a former provincial Progressive Conservative politician, Health Minister and Treasurer, who was in private consulting practice, and two administrators from British Columbia, neither of whom had much experience in paediatric issues. The lack of experience in paediatric issues was not seen as important at the outset, as it was predicted that the major closures would affect the adult hospitals. The Hyndman Group reviewed the Price Waterhouse report and heard the comments of all the boards, then recommended that there be only three hospital sites in Calgary – Foothills, Rockyview and Peter Lougheed. The Alberta Children's Hospital was to close and its in-patient services be transferred to Foothills Hospital.[10] Despite the obvious involvement of the government in the choice of procedure and consultants, the Premier tried to distance himself from the recommendations by saying this was "not the government's report, but commissioned by local hospital boards."[11]

An analysis of the findings indicated a lack of understanding of paediatric services overall and suggested that planning was for in-patient services alone, without attention to ambulatory care or in-patient–ambulatory co-operation. The Hyndman Group did not see the need for specific and special services for children in laboratories, X-ray, emergency department, operating room, and so on. They saw them as expensive duplication, whereas parents, public and paediatric health caregivers saw them as meeting distinct needs and providing good value for money.

The Hyndman Report was made public on April 13, 1994, and produced a strong reaction, with the public responding in a way that was clear, emotional and powerful. There were public rallies[12] at the Alberta Children's Hospital and the "Blue Ribbon Campaign" developed. A parent placed a blue ribbon on her lapel and encouraged others to follow her example to indicate support for the hospital. Supportive letters, phone calls and faxes were sent to each and every public figure, including MLAs, government ministers and the Premier. Public contact with politicians on this one issue was greater than on any other single issue in the history of the Progressive Conservative government. The protests received by the government were overwhelmingly in favor of retention of the Alberta Children's Hospital at its present site and in its present format. Staff at the Alberta Children's Hospital were in support, but were seen by the government as "a special interest group," a phrase used to designate any group of individuals knowledgeable on an issue. Personal job losses, although feared by some, were not a large issue, as most of the professional staff would be transferred to wherever the new paediatric facility would be developed, in the same way as there had been transfers in 1982 from Foothills Hospital to the Alberta Children's Hospital. Most of the staff were determined to keep the hospital because they were convinced that it was best for children. A few staff wished the issue to be over, whatever the result, as the uncertainty was stressful. Some wished for a move to the Foothills to be nearer the academic centre. Black humor abounded and, perversely, helped.

The public did not fully believe that the Alberta Children's Hospital would close. So extreme was the anxiety that rumors appeared and disappeared. One persistent rumor was that the closure of the Alberta Children's Hospital was a ruse and the government would suddenly announce that it would not close and in the midst of public support for this move would be able to close the Holy Cross and the Calgary General hospitals without opposition. The Alberta Children's Hospital and the other hospitals were reviewing the options presented by Hyndman at the same time as the public protests were continuing. There were detailed cost analyses and a study of the move's impact on quality of care. The cost of converting part of Foothills Hospital (the Special Services Building) to make it suitable for children was prohibitive and the premises would be less desirable than the 17th Avenue building. Most involved in paediatric care felt that if $90 million (the sum mentioned) was available, there were many priorities before the replacement of a building built specifically for paediatric health care and in good condition. There might have been some improvement in the quality of care of a minority of children with a great loss in quality of care for the overwhelming majority. These reports[13] were said to influence the Minister more than the political protest.

The response of the Alberta Children's Hospital Board during the whole process was paradoxical. Members of the Board did have an interest in child health but were government appointees and motivated to reduce health-care costs. The Alberta Children's Hospital Board members may have shown support privately to their political friends and acquaintances, but they were not visible when the public was showing support. The Alberta Children's Hospital Foundation took the neutral position that its role was to fund child health care, and it was the government's decision where that would be provided. The Children's Hospital Aid Society (CHAS), on the other hand, lobbied actively for the retention of the Alberta Children's Hospital.

The Calgary Regional Health Authority, which now had authority over ACH, had to consider many projects which had been placed "on hold" by the previous board. One was the provision of a cardiac catheterization laboratory at the Alberta Children's Hospital, the top priority since 1990. This project had been supported by the other acute-care hospitals in Calgary, approved by the Department of Health, but had not been approved by the Alberta Children's Hospital Board, despite the fact that building costs were to be provided by the Alberta Children's Hospital Foundation and the CHAS. This lack of approval was an example of the Board's extreme caution and its equivocal response to the survival of the hospital. When this issue reached the new Calgary Regional Health Authority, a bureaucrat reviewed the proposal and his suggested rejection (without discussion with clinicians at the Alberta Children's Hospital) was supported by senior medical authorities. However, the Calgary Regional Health Authority insisted on a full re-evaluation, approved the proposal, and what is now called the Special Procedures Room opened in November 1996. Another paediatric issue to be dealt with by the Calgary Regional Health Authority was the placement of paediatric beds. Following public consultation, beds were maintained at the Peter Lougheed Centre, but the beds at the Rockyview Hospital were transferred to the Alberta Children's Hospital.[14]

The major struggle in 1994 illustrated clearly different views and attitudes about children's hospitals in general. Parents who are users of the various children's hospitals in Canada and the paediatric caregivers within them consider these hospitals not only to be important but truly to be general hospitals for children. By having a children's hospital as a focus for health-care delivery, many professionals can dedicate their careers to children and improve their expertise in health-care delivery to children. Many support services, such as low-dose radiation and microsampling of blood, were provided in children's hospitals long before they received general acceptance. Children's hospitals have in common a desire to develop outreach services and have been proponents and advocates of the development of home care. Parental pressure has been the major factor in these trends, but children's hospitals have tried to make it easy for the parent's point of view to be heard, and in Calgary the Community Advisory Committee has been strongly supported by the Alberta Children's Hospital Board and the hospital's administration. The linking of in-patients, ambulatory care, emergency, day care and the school, which has been a feature of care at the Alberta Children's Hospital, has been highly successful in the provision of a high level of care to children, without incurring undue expense. Yet, despite these advantages noted by consumers and professionals alike, many health-care bureaucrats and administrators still do not support the concept of a children's hospital. The move to incorporate in-patient units for children into general hospitals, without providing separate paediatric facilities in ambulatory care, radiology, emergency and so on, persists. The need for special facilities for children is conceded by all, but the value of a close geographic relation of the various components of paediatric services is not understood by those not engaged in the care of children. The struggle between protagonists and antagonists of children's hospitals will continue, as this is an issue which requires constant re-examination. Some high-technology developments may be too expensive to provide specifically for children and, in many areas, the population is too small to justify the cost of a separate facility for children financially. However, wherever care for children is delivered, it is always better to be in premises with their needs in mind, by professionals skilled in paediatric care and under the control of an administration dedicated to the best interests of children and their caregivers. ❖

References

1. Calgary Regional Health Authority and Alberta Health, News release. July 14, 1994.
2. *Report: Child Health Services in Alberta: A Provincial Model.* November, 1993.
3. O'Handley, Kathryn, ed. *The Canadian Parliamentary Guide.* Globe and Mail Publication, Toronto, 1993, p. 525.
4. Normandin, Pierre G., ed. *The Canadian Parliamentary Guide.* Ottawa, 1972, p. 498.
5. Don Martin. *The Calgary Herald*, April 16, 1994, p. A3.
6. *Alberta's Debt and Deficit.* Workbook of the Director of Communication, Alberta Treasury, 1993.
7. Data provided by Finance Department, CRHA, April 1996.
8. Terms of Reference, Calgary Acute Care Services Planning Study. June 19, 1993.
9. Calgary Regional Acute Care Planning Study – Acute Care Restructuring Discussion Document Final Report. January 1994.
10. Report of the Facilitation Group on Health Services in Calgary, Alberta. April 11, 1994.
11. *The Calgary Herald*, April 15, 1994, p. A2.
12. *The Calgary Herald*, April 15, 1994, p. F11, and April 16, 1994, p. A1.
13. Alberta Children's Hospital Task Force: Quality of Care Subcommittee. Final Report. May 26, 1994; Capital Cost Working Group. Final Report. May 25, 1994.
14. Paediatric Community Health Task Force. Report and Recommendations to the Calgary Regional Health Authority. September 7, 1995.

Family Experiences

The number of children treated at the Alberta Children's Hospital in the last sixteen years so outnumbers those treated in any previous epoch of the Alberta Children's Hospital that it is difficult to pick a few experiences to represent so many. In addition, in previous sections of the book, we dealt with patient memories, but in today's hospital children no longer spend many years as in-patients. Now children are admitted to the hospital for brief periods for a specific treatment, even if they have life-threatening and complicated illnesses, and then looked after at home. Often they return to the DAT Centre or for further brief admissions. We will describe the experience of only a few children, who usually have had contact with many different areas. We have not described the experience of families who bring their child on only one occasion to the Emergency Department or for one brief admission to the hospital or Day Surgery, not because we do not think these services are important. The expressions of gratitude when families leave the hospital attest to the quality of care given, whether admission was long or short.

Charlie was born on January 3, 1982, and his mother recognized that there was something wrong right from the moment of birth, but the maternity unit staff told her she was over-reacting and that he was a lazy baby. Eventually Charlie was transferred to the Alberta Children's Hospital for observation. Not much later, the parents were called at midnight to be told that Charlie was being transferred to the Paediatric Intensive Care Unit at Foothills Hospital because of blue spells. The parents were alarmed, but also optimistic as it looked as if Charlie was now going to get help. A surgeon was consulted, as was a neurologist from the Alberta Children's Hospital, and it turned out that Charlie had a form of muscular dystrophy. Once the Intensive Care Unit opened at the Alberta Children's Hospital, Charlie was transferred back. In spite of her frustration and anxiety, his mother felt supported by the doctors and nurses.

The family was now finding out the Alberta Children's Hospital was more than just a hospital, and in the DAT Centre many caring people would take Charlie's two-year-old brother Justin for hours while mom and dad met with doctors and nurses. Over the weeks of the first admission, Charlie had the first of many surgeries, and the odds were never in his favor. Throughout his many operations, physicians and nurses from different specialties co-ordinated his care. His life consisted of periods of recovery at home interspersed with periods of treatment at the hospital. The hospital became his second home, a place where he made friends and felt secure and happy.

At two-and-a-half years of age, Charlie was enrolled at the Gordon Townsend School in the multi-handicap program. This seemed to be the first step in the beginning of a new life. His mother was with Charlie for a couple of weeks to help the staff understand Charlie's needs, and it was easier for his mother to leave him knowing that all of Charlie's physicians were nearby.

When Charlie was four years old, he started kindergarten, then later entered grade one. It was felt that Charlie would benefit from an electric wheelchair, and he turned out to be the youngest student to master this equipment. He began playing wheelchair floor hockey in the gym at the school and became a member of the Townsend Tigers and then a member of the Saturday Wheelchair Floor Hockey League. Charlie excelled in this and became one of the stars. Charlie's two burning desires were to meet Michael Jackson and to go to Disneyland. The Children's Wish Foundation was able to provide a trip to Disneyland, where Charlie and his brother Justin had the time of their

life, a time the family still remembers. Charlie's health deteriorated, as is expected with the condition he had, but his parents always had support from the hospital staff and felt that all the staff took the time to be patient and explained what was happening to him. He died at home, as he had wished, on February 26, 1995.

Many children with chronic diseases attend the Alberta Children's Hospital. Many continue to require special medical care as adults. There may be an abrupt transition to an adult hospital, but all of those we have spoken to have warm memories of the care they received at the Alberta Children's Hospital. There is a small group of adults who continue to attend the Alberta Children's Hospital, mainly those with hemophilia. Some of them even prefer to come to the Alberta Children's Hospital Emergency Department rather than the adult emergency department, as they feel the staff are familiar with their condition and give them quick and efficient treatment.

Children with cancer have different memories. We spoke to two patients, Christopher and Shannon, both diagnosed in the late 1980s. Cancer care had been centralized with the opening of the Tom Baker Cancer Centre just before ACH opened. Thus in-patient and out-patient care for children and adults was at the Foothills site. However, the in-patient ward for children with cancer opened at ACH in 1982 and as the out-patient clinic remained at the Tom Baker Cancer Centre, children and parents faced a tough situation. For example, if during a visit to the clinic at the Tom Baker Cancer Centre it was decided that the child would have to be admitted, he or she had to go home, pack and go the Alberta Children's Hospital for admission. This was a problem for parents who lived far away. Now, if admission is needed, the child simply stays in the hospital after the out-patient visit, and his or her things are brought along later.

Their memories of the clinic at the Tom Baker Cancer Centre are of a long, dark corridor with some chairs against one side and a huge fish tank at the end the only diversion. There was one small playroom with a box of toys and one chair, and anyone who wanted to talk to the children had to sit on the floor.

If a medical procedure was performed, the patient was moved back to the hallway afterwards to stay there until he/she could leave. On procedure day, many children were violently sick all the time in the hallway, and this was obviously frightening for the other children waiting. Waiting was a reality, as the physicians had to go back and forth between the two hospitals, and so if an emergency arose, the out-patients at Tom Baker Cancer Centre had to wait for the physician to travel back to the Alberta Children's Hospital to deal with it.

The nurses and technicians felt that it was not fair for children to have cancer and these thoughts made it hard for them to deal with the children. The children themselves found it difficult to be in the same area as adults with cancer. In the hallway, the children liked to play and have a wheelchair race, whereas the adults had a preference for peace and quiet. Neither party was happy. There were also advantages in this situation: it was easier to get together with other patients and plan the day starting with arrival time around coffee, tea and juice carts which would be wheeled around by volunteers. However, after coffee and juice, it was difficult to pass time waiting, because the waiting area was too small to bring a brother or sister as a companion.

Despite all these issues, the care offered at the clinic was considered good. Shannon and Christopher felt that there were only two physicians who knew everything about them, compared with now when they have to repeat everything to the many people involved. Moreover, they both remembered the small knitted finger puppets that came with pokes, and they often ended up with whole families of these puppets.

However, both Shannon and Christopher felt the move to the Alberta Children's Hospital in 1991 was a vast improvement. There was full integration of the Paediatric Oncology Program, and it was much easier to be optimistic and positive. They remember it as "stepping into the daylight." The new out-patient oncology area is large with bright colors, and in fact some of the children were intimidated at first by the brightness and openness. The play lady came for crafts and games and managed to bring back the group feeling, helped by cookies from the cafeteria. The atmosphere at the Alberta Children's Hospital lends itself to laughter.

Lesley, the last patient discussed here, was born in 1990. She was diagnosed with a blood disorder some years later. In this disorder (elliptocytosis), the blood cells are broken down rapidly, there are episodes of jaundice and the spleen becomes enlarged. The spleen usually has to be removed once it reaches a large size.

In 1996, it was time to remove Lesley's spleen, and traditional surgery would have meant a long operation. Her abdomen would be opened, the spleen identified and carefully removed. There is a new technique called laparoscopic surgery that was first used in adults but is being increasingly used in children. In this technique, anaesthesia is still used, but the surgeon makes two or three small incisions and inserts a small telescope and instruments through the incisions. With the telescope, the area requiring surgery can be seen, and much of the surgery can be carried out through the small incisions. The spleen itself was removed through a slightly bigger incision in the abdomen. Lesley's surgery was May 6, 1996, and she was discharged on May 13, back at school within two weeks and playing T-ball within three weeks.

Many different memories could have been included, but we have illustrated just a few facets of care through these stories of experiences at the Alberta Children's Hospital. These patients have one thing in common: they have all benefited from Alberta Children's Hospital with the support from all the staff and organization as well as its commitment to the latest technology.

PART SEVEN

CONSTANTS IN THE LIFE OF THE HOSPITAL

❖❖❖❖❖❖❖❖❖❖❖❖❖

The School and the Alberta Children's Hospital

The south entrance of the hospital dominates 20th Street, and the yellow school buses there in the morning and afternoon are a sure sign that this is a school. Education has always been an integral part of the hospital. Nevertheless, the school, while part of the hospital, has its own identity.

Over the years, the school clientele has changed considerably. At first, the students were all long-term in-patients and attended for months and years. Now students may be in- or out-patients and have intensive treatment and rehabilitation combined into education, and attend for short periods as preparation for integration with their local school. The teachers have also changed from non-certified teachers to certified professionals working within an interdisciplinary team.

Why was education part of the first hospital and still present today? Schooling is a large part of the normal life of all children and is also a true morale builder. Mastering new tasks and ideas helps sick children to focus on their abilities, instead of on their disabilities. Many of the children had difficulty in physical activities, and developing their mental abilities was particularly important as was building their self-esteem. Schooling involved general knowledge as well as teaching skills that could form the basis for further education and jobs.

Long-term hospitalization meant going to the hospital school, so patients would not be behind their peers and would be able to fit in on return to the local school. Moreover, as one of the matrons was fond of pointing out, the child who has had to struggle with acceptance of a disease is often better equipped to deal with problems and demands in life later on.

The first teacher, Miss Clarke, started her work immediately as the first hospital opened in 1922, but her appointment was temporary. The

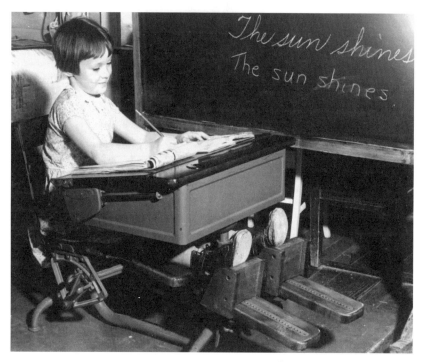

Child at special desk.

government issued a grant toward the teacher's salary of $750[1] thus acknowledging the importance of education for children in the hospital. There is no specific mention of the teacher's actual salary in the early hospital reports, since these costs were part of, and absorbed in, the running of the hospital. The matron of the hospital was not only responsible for the nurses but also for other personnel including teachers. The Board of the hospital hired people based on her recommendations.

Then Mabel Mappin, previously teaching at Brickburn House, was hired. Her formal assignment was teaching as well as supervising crafts. The success of the flower and handicraft industry, a vital component of the rehabilitation program, was certainly due to her initiative and enterprise.[2] In 1928, the sale of paper flowers netted $600, a substantial amount of money at that time.[3]

In 1937, Fran McClure (née Dande) was interviewed by Florence Reid, the hospital matron. She remained the only teacher for five years and stayed at the school a total of thirty years. Patients at the hospital became "her" children. When she got married, several of the children attended her wedding as guests. After the ceremony, she and her husband drove up to the hospital to see the other children before leaving her bouquet of red roses with them.[4]

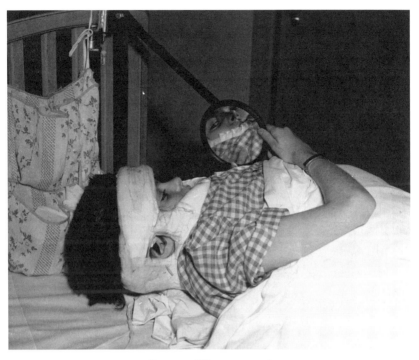

"I can still see you."

The provincial correspondence courses (grades one to twelve) were the basis of education at this time. Children who had repeated admissions to the hospital could continue their course work either at home, local school or in the hospital. The teachers would either work with the pupils in a classroom, sometimes in specially adapted desks or, if they could not be carried up and down the stairs, the teacher would go to their bedside. Working with the patients could be quite challenging. Some youngsters lying in traction or in a total body cast were linked to the world only by mirrors. As late as 1958, there was a report by a teacher describing a child in her classroom. This boy "… was rigid in an all-encompassing body cast that covered him from head to thigh, with openings for his hair, face, ears and arms, flat on his stomach with pillows under his elbows and a hand mirror to reflect what was going on around him. I began to pamper him by omitting his turn from the blackboard accuracy drill. But twice around the room, calling on all but him, he asked me for a turn. By adjusting his mirror he could watch the clock face of numbers on the blackboard, and before the period was over, he was the winner in the contest for speed."[5]

In 1932, the school was officially established under the Department of Education and thereby qualified for a government grant. The teaching

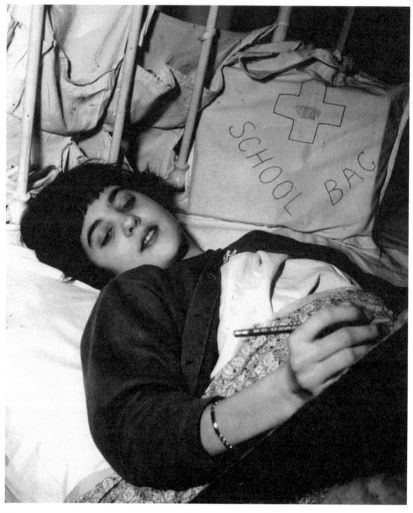

Special school bag.

staff recommended by the school board now had to be certified. By the time the second hospital closed (in 1951), there were three teachers. High-school students were still enrolled in the correspondence course and wrote their final exams within the regular time frame. Fitting in teaching periods with medical rounds and visits, physiotherapy, brace fitting, nursing and housekeeping procedures was no easy task and reflected the necessary co-operation with the hospital staff. Children who could move around went to the classroom, but many were still taught in the wards. Each bed had an easel table that could easily be adjusted. Children each had a school bag for pencils, crayons and books, a heavy white cotton bag with

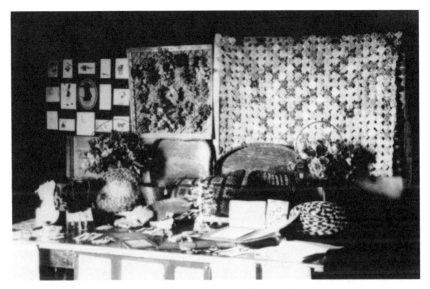

Handicrafts made by the patients.

a red cross on the front and the child's name printed on white tape. Hung on metal hooks below the beds at the end of the day, school bags were instantly available for the next day. Nowadays parents or classmates sometimes bring in homework assignments from regular schools. Apart from their schoolwork, the children also had occupational therapy and enjoyed learning and making many different crafts.

One of the patients in 1941 was Bill. He had spastic paralysis, and when at home, his sisters used to pull him in his wagon. This meant going to school only when it was sunny, definitely never in winter. When he became a resident of the Junior Red Cross Children's Hospital at age thirteen, he was placed in grade five. Depending on his physical ability that day, he would either use his walking sticks to get to the third-floor classroom, or the teacher would come to his bedside. There was no elevator in this building nor were the hallways wide enough to accommodate wheelchairs. Bill felt so much at home in the hospital that, like any other normal child, he would get into mischief and distinctly remembers being called into the office. His favorite activities were woodcarving, leather tooling and basket weaving. He still displays some of his handiwork in his home. As Bill showed expertise in these skills, he often returned as a volunteer during later summers to teach other patients the skills he had learned. To this day, he still works in his well-equipped workshop behind his home. He certainly embodies the philosophy of the hospital that patients can become self-sufficient.[6]

In June 1946, the school was renamed the Alberta Children's Hospital School, and the Calgary Public School Board assumed full responsibility

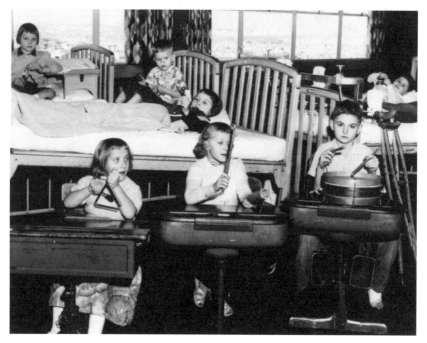

Band.

for the teachers and educational programs, with more focus on academic subjects. Fridays were still set aside as handicraft day. Many volunteers were actively involved in the different programs in the school, for example, knitting, crocheting, leather tooling, rug making, shell work, embroidery and music. The younger children were charmed by a retired elementary teacher who went from ward to ward telling fairy stories. Once every two weeks was letter-writing day, when children wrote a letter to their parents, assisted by volunteers. This was a must, since it was the only way that parents were certain to receive word from their children.[7]

There were also volunteers who came to play the piano and organized a rhythm band with the children. Janet Warren, recognized as an accomplished church organist and choir director, was one of them. Her comment when she was asked to volunteer at the hospital was, "I am not sure that I can work with sick children within a hospital setting." She began in 1948 with the idea that she would at least give it a try. Thirteen years later, she was still there volunteering. Every Tuesday afternoon, she would either teach singing to children who could come to the third floor where the piano was, or she would go around the hospital with her box of rhythm instruments and a tuning fork. During her years as a volunteer, there were students who made an unforgettable impression on her and vice versa. One was a personable, bright young lad who always wanted

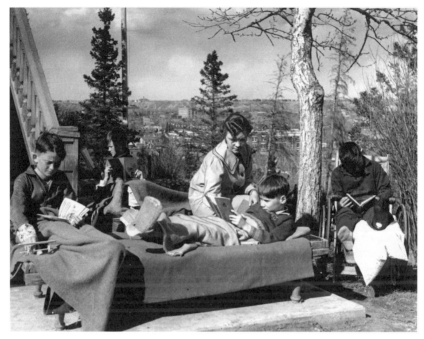

School outside.

to play the drums, but this was next to impossible with his twisted hands and feet. But persist he did, to such an extent that, a few years later, Janet happened to see and hear him play with a musical group. Another student Janet remembers was a teenager in a full body cast. She told Janet not to bother coming to her bedside because she could not sing a note. When they met again, some years later at the Crescent Heights Library, she told Janet that she was now a member of the High School Glee Club and had made singing part of her life.[8]

The move to the present site (the third hospital) meant welcome changes in the facility as well as the school program. There was now much more space, with one room totally devoted to speech therapy and another for occupational therapy. There was also an administration area including the principal's office and a staff room for the teachers and volunteers. Three large classrooms with glare-proof blackboards, indirect lighting and desks specially modified for orthopaedic patients completed the facility. Indeed some of the teaching was even done outside on the sundeck. Handicrafts became an evening activity where copper pictures and clay work took the place of weaving and other crafts.

In 1953, the Alberta Children's Hospital School was described as among the best in the country by the Department of Education. That year, the school had five full-time teachers, two volunteer teachers, three music teachers, five storytellers, six letter-writers and twenty handicraft teachers. An education department official stated in his report, "I do not know of any school anywhere that achieves its purpose more fully."[9] The report continued, "... services at the hospital school cannot be estimated in ordinary terms. Actually the feeling of achievement and the self confidence it inspires in pupils, is a very important part of the whole rehabilitation program."

This can best be illustrated by an example from the report, *Beds and Blackboards*, where the teacher describes her shock at finding a memo on her desk on Monday morning that J. is not coming to school, because his leg had been amputated and he could not be moved to the classroom yet. "However he would like to see you." She describes visiting J. in his bed,

> ... *his face drained of colour, the blanket flatter on the left where his leg had been amputated. He smiled and asked me* ... *"What page are the children on in arithmetic? I do not want them to get too far ahead of me...."* *By Wednesday, he was back in the classroom and when discharged at Christmas, he was leading his classmates in arithmetic, spelling and language.*[10]

In September 1962, the school officially came under the jurisdiction of the Calgary Public School Board which, until then, had only been responsible for the salary of the teachers. This meant further reorganization, and, as a result, correspondence courses had limited use as supplemental teaching material.

In the 1970s, there was public controversy about the safety of the school. After the move of the Cerebral Palsy Clinic, space had become a real problem, and by 1974, the school was housed in trailers. There was a major concern that the school was unsafe and unsanitary.[11] The provincial government was accused of gross negligence and irresponsibility. A school trustee called the school "a mice-infested firetrap." There was also a growing concern with gas leaks from the furnaces that heated the temporary buildings. There was no nurse's room, and washrooms were inadequate. This controversial situation no doubt had a positive effect on the speed of the planning and completion of the new school. The Minister of Education at that time was Lou Hyndman, who, later, as a private consultant, recommended closure of the Alberta Children's Hospital in 1994. In December 1977, the first stage of the new Child Health Centre, the $2.3 million school, officially opened. The new building boasted twelve large classrooms. The gymnasium accommodated recreational activities, as well as doubling as an area for dining and school assemblies. The corridors were wider than usual to facilitate the movement of wheelchairs and beds. After a contest for a new name, the Alberta Children's Hospital School was officially renamed the Dr. Gordon Townsend School in July 1978.

In 1979, many of the students of the Dr. Gordon Townsend School

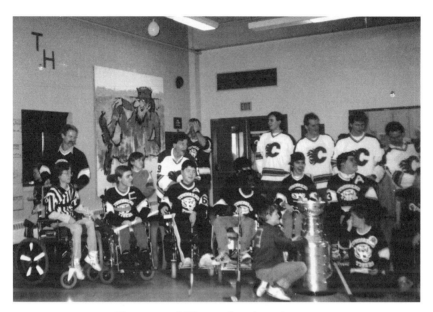

Townsend Tigers hockey team.

became actively involved in the movie business. The movie *Touched by Love*, based on the book, was filmed in Banff with sixteen pupils of the school participating in a variety of roles. The movie was based on a true story of a young girl abandoned by her parents at birth when they find out she is handicapped. She becomes withdrawn and only blossoms during a correspondence with Elvis Presley. The students were all housed at the Banff Springs Hotel for three weeks, something to remember for many years.[12]

However, the movie business was not everyday life at school. The school day was as normal as possible based on the individual needs of the children. For example, it was often necessary to incorporate other disciplines such as swimming, speech and physiotherapy into school activities. One of the memorable programs that assisted integration back into society was the tuck shop. This was an initiative started and operated by entrepreneurs, who happened to be youngsters with disabilities. The hospital carpenter helped them to get started by building a display counter that was easily accessible from a wheelchair. The Tuck Shop sold a little of everything, even ice cream kept cool in a donated freezer. The two executives were Arlene (fourteen years old) and David (fifteen years old). They involved as many as seventeen youngsters paid by the hour. They were both in wheelchairs but that certainly did not keep them from operating a profitable business. In six months, they had made a net profit of $300.[13]

The School Board and Hospital Board worked closely together to provide and create the atmosphere that was conducive to these kinds of initiatives. There was a delicate balance of responsibilities and financial

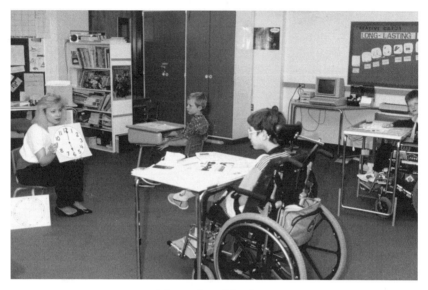

The school today.

management between those two boards. The School Board was responsible for the education side of the school, including teachers and curriculum. The hospital was responsible for everything else, for example, the building, child-care workers, therapy, nursing staff and cleaning staff. One issue is an example of the complex relationship between the Alberta Children's Hospital and the School Board. Child-care workers were employed by the hospital and were well known to the children and parents. The hospital dismissed all of them in 1993 in response to funding cuts, and similar care was then provided to the children by classroom assistants, hired by the School Board under different conditions of employment. The hospital reimbursed the School Board for expenses, and overall several hundred thousand dollars were saved each year. There was extreme anxiety when the change was announced, reflecting the high level of emotional involvement on both sides.

The ultimate aim is to integrate the children in a community school as soon as possible. There are criteria to ensure that the Dr. Gordon Townsend School does not duplicate other services available in Calgary and southern Alberta. At the present time, the population of the Dr. Gordon Townsend School may be grouped into one of the following categories: acute rehabilitation for students who require intensive individualized therapy following trauma or surgery, brain-injured students who require intensive therapy in the cognitive and physical realm, medically fragile students who require acute or chronic care combined with a modified educational program, mental health students and in-patients.

Although the school population has changed over the years, the philosophy is unchanged. The thrust is to provide education and treatment to students who, for reasons of physical, emotional or developmental disability, require a specialized, safe and therapeutic environment.❖

References

1. *Minutes*. Canadian Red Cross Society, Alberta Division, November 14, 1922.
2. *Annual Report*. Canadian Red Cross Society, Alberta Division, 1923, p. 13.
3. *Annual Report*. Canadian Red Cross Society, Alberta Division, 1928, p. 34.
4. F. McClure, personal communication.
5. Williams, Marian. *Beds and Blackboards*. Undated report, p. 3.
6. Bill, personal communication.
7. *Annual Report*. Canadian Red Cross Society, Alberta Division, 1949, pp. 65, 66.
8. Janet Warren, personal communication.
9. *The Calgary Herald*, June 22, 1953.
10. Williams, Marian. *Beds and Blackboards*. pp. 2–3.
11. *The Calgary Herald*, February 23, 1974.
12. *The Calgary Herald*, November 3, 1979.
13. *The Calgary Herald*, August 2, 1977.

Further reading

MacBeath, R. An examination of the Programs/Therapies at the Dr. Gordon Townsend School, using the Alternative School's Concept of Education, 1987.

McDonald, H.M. "The Place of a School in a Children's Hospital." *Medical Journal of Australia*. November 29, 1969, pp. 1108–1112.

Alberta Children's Hospital, Program Inventory, December 16, 1992.

Dr. Gordon Townsend School, Staff Handbook, 1996–97.

Support Staff – Always There

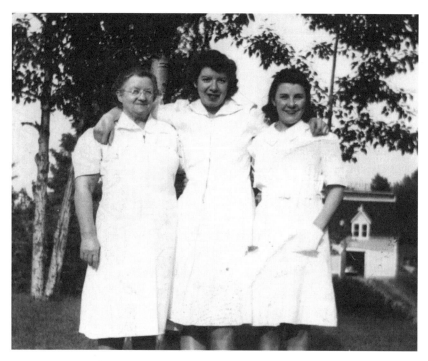

Cook and waitresses in the second hospital.

The support staff are essential to the smooth running of the hospital but by and large are unrecognized because physicians, nurses and other health-care professionals are more visible. At the Alberta Children's Hospital, the support staff tend to be very devoted to the children and keen to ensure that high standards are maintained.

These include the staff involved with housekeeping and catering, maintenance staff whose help is eagerly sought when there is a problem, porters, secretaries, receptionists, switchboard operators, parking attendants, security and so on. Who does not know the porter going around the hospital with candies? If this gentleman sees any member of staff looking unhappy, he hands over a candy, receiving a smile in response.

"HR" are the initials of both Health Records and Human Resources. The modern Health Records Department not only stores patient records (and retrieves them when needed) but also prepares a summary of the work of the hospital. Letters and notes must be typed and dictation can be sent by phone to the transcriptionist who produces documents at high speed. Human Resources deals with all aspects of employment and is often the first contact a new employee has with the hospital.

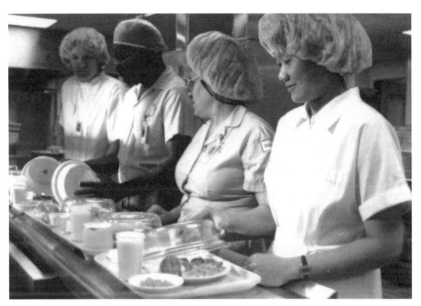

Preparing food.

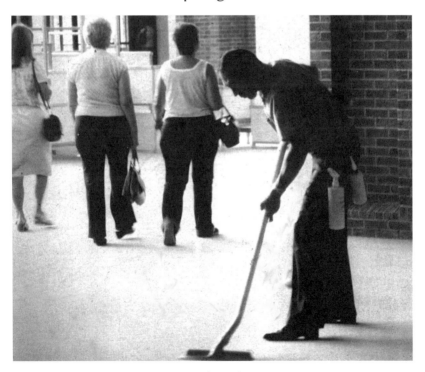

Housekeeping.

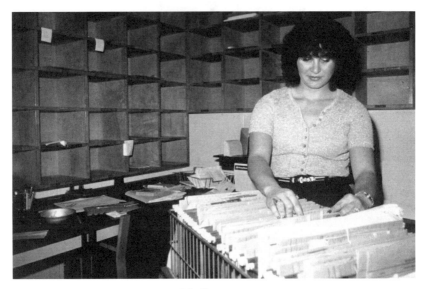

Mail room.

One of the support areas that is often overlooked is the power plant, which has always been part of the hospital. Previously it was under the East Annex in a tunnel between the hospital and the annex. In the late 1970s, it was rebuilt to allow for the new buildings, including the Dr. Gordon Townsend School. The new section opened in 1982, with power concentrated at one point in the hospital, new boilers, new freezers, a new system for central steam heating and water and also air conditioning and ventilation control. Trained engineers can shut down parts and monitor fire alarms and know when there are problems with electricity, although they do not deal with them themselves. In general, many of the maintenance staff believe that it is better to operate in a businesslike way, though they recognize that the larger organization is more bureaucratic and less personal.

Even though we cannot mention all of their different functions, the support staff are an essential part of the hospital, one of the ingredients that creates its distinct character.❖

Volunteers – Essential to Hospital Growth

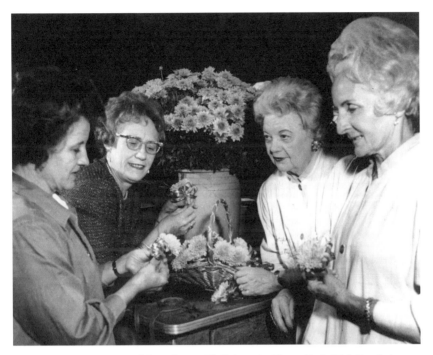

Boutonniere–making bee, Children's Hospital Aid Society.

Volunteers are an integral part of any hospital and particularly important in the Alberta Children's Hospital. Volunteers played a major role in starting the hospital, continued to be important throughout the history of the hospital and remain essential today. This is one area where it is easy to miss important people; there are so many different volunteers who contribute so much now and have done so in the past, most often without a desire for recognition. The popularity of this commitment is shown by the long waiting list to join the volunteer group.

A wide range of individuals are included under the title "volunteer," all of whom supplement hospital services and act as ambassadors. Some volunteers are part of the official Volunteer Service and have training for specific functions, others work at home preparing, for example, clothing for children, still others work within other organizations that help the Alberta Children's Hospital, and, finally, many work to raise funds for the hospital and for the Alberta Children's Hospital Foundation. Many are involved in volunteering for the hospital in more than one way. The staff themselves are often so devoted that they volunteer their time for extra activities at the hospital.

The early volunteers included the Junior Red Cross Society, Kinsmen, Children's Hospital Aid Society, many businesses in Calgary and rural Alberta, the Active 20/30 Club, the radio station co-ordinating live broadcasts, Shriners and many different lodges, clubs, organizations and individuals. Many of these continue their volunteer activities for the hospital. Of these many groups, two have been part of the hospital from the beginning and continue to provide strong support today, namely the Children's Hospital Aid Society and the Kinsmen Club.

The Children's Hospital Aid Society started in 1908 as the Women's Hospital Aid Society of the General Hospital and thus precedes the Alberta Children's Hospital. The secretary of this committee called a meeting of young girls to form an auxiliary to the parent society with Jean Pinkham as the first President. The auxiliary was designated to look after the children's ward, and by 1910 the auxiliary had grown as large as the parent body. Twelve of the older married women left the organization and started the Young Women's Benevolent Society under J.H. Woods which changed its name to the Samaritan Club.[1] The Girls' Auxiliary was incorporated as the Girls' Hospital Aid Society in 1910 and, a day after the Junior Red Cross Children's Hospital opened in 1922, became a corporate society, under the leadership of Edythe Lillie. By 1926, the members felt that they should have a name change; the original group had stayed together and were thus rather older "girls" and also felt the word "children" should be included as being appropriate for this work. From 1926 onwards, this dedicated group of women has been known as the Children's Hospital Aid Society.

The contribution of the Children's Hospital Aid Society over the years has been outstanding, and it is difficult to pick out any one donation. For example, in 1936, $2,695 was donated for the maintenance of a ten-bed ward, and, in fact, members of the CHAS visited the ward and got to know the children.[2] That money was raised many different ways, including selling tickets at rugby games, rain or shine, hail or snow, in the fall each year for thirty-five years.

There were many innovative fundraiser programs. For example, in 1942, horse show program sales started, and members also raffled a house that they had bought themselves. At this time, however, the members realized that one large fundraising project might make better use of their efforts than many smaller intensive fundraisers. Two members suggested starting the Easter Seal campaign after receiving seals in their mail from the United States. In 1946, the first Crippled Children's Easter Seal Campaign raised a whopping $4,761.69 from a small mail-out to a limited number of known individuals and businesses. Within eight years, this grew to over $23,000, all of which was turned over to the Alberta Red Cross Crippled Children's Hospital. The first Easter Seal party for all the children and their parents was in 1946. This particular campaign is now a nationwide event run in conjunction with the Alberta Rehabilitation Council for the Disabled.

The CHAS retained its focus, but with the coming of government financing of hospitals in the late 1950s, its role was not clear. The Alberta Children's Hospital Board felt that, as far as the CHAS was concerned, it was "not now in need of funds."[3] At that time, the CHAS thought that it would devote itself to special cases, helping with school costs and donating money to other worthwhile causes involving children.

The prediction that the CHAS was not needed was incredibly wide of the mark. In all, the CHAS has donated well over $2 million to the Alberta Children's Hospital, always for specific projects, and contributed extensively, for example, to the hospital library, swimming pool, Child Abuse Centre, and the DAT Centre, along with seventeen handi-buses over many years. Some of the recent contributions include the helipad and Special Procedures Room, items essential for a tertiary-care hospital.

Now the CHAS raises a significant portion of its donations through the annual golf tournament which started in 1983. In 1984, the gift shop, Emily's Window, opened, with two members of the CHAS on the organizing committee and several other CHAS members involved as volunteers. Ten years later, the profit from the shop was $60,000.

Another organization that has contributed extensively to the Alberta Children's Hospital over the years is the Kinsmen Club, which is dedicated to fellowship and service among businessmen between twenty-one and forty years of age. The Kinsmen Club of Calgary was formed in 1924 following the lead of clubs in other cities in Canada, and in 1926, one of the members strongly recommended involvement in the Junior Red Cross Children's Hospital. Three weeks after that recommendation, the Kinsmen had organized their first birthday party, for which each member purchased a gift for "his" child at the hospital. From then on, every Saturday, four or five Kinsmen would take the children out for a car ride and also took on the responsibility of taking them to the Stampede.

By 1931, they had been involved in donating orthopaedic equipment, establishing a library and also making sure that the children enjoyed a circus program. The Kinsmen organized Christmas parties and gave up Christmas morning with their own families to be in the hospital. By 1937, CFCN radio began broadcasting the party so that patients could send greetings to their family members at home. The Kinsmen continued to work at the Junior Red Cross Children's Hospital throughout World War II, and, even though gasoline was severely rationed, the Saturday drives were continued.

The Kinsmen had started a "Mile of Dimes" to provide powdered milk for children in Britain during the war, which continued after the war but became a fundraiser for the Alberta Children's Hospital. In 1946, a station wagon was donated to transport children back and forth to other

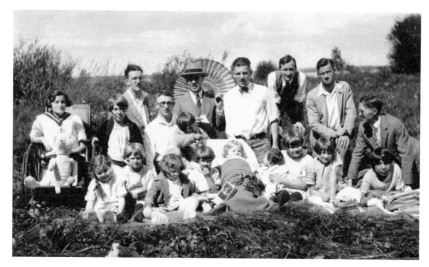

Kinsmen and kids in the country.

hospitals for operations. The car came to an unfortunate demise when, during a Kinsmen conference, it was filled up with cement!

The Kinsmen were instrumental in the realization of the Alberta Children's Hospital Research Centre and continue to support it through the Kinsmen Annual Lottery, which started in 1974. To honor their contribution, this part of the hospital is called The Kinsmen Research Centre.

A snapshot of volunteer activities at a point in time (1966) shows a wide range of functions.[4] For example, the Kinsmen worked in kindergarten in the preschool program, operated a snack bar on orthopaedic outpatient days, and often participated in the evening in crafts, movies, singing, Scouts, Guides, Brownies and Cubs. At that time, there were eighty volunteers, who wore mauve and white checked uniforms. In the summer, to allow the adults to have time off, fifty teens called Candy Stripers appeared in pink and white to take over their duties. Other special groups included the ladies helping sew linen and clothes, the Jaycees assisting in the Friday movie, the Kinsmen organizing the Saturday drive and providing parties, the Junior League of Calgary who helped in the orthopaedic out-patient clinic, entertainment groups, and the CHAS "who always helped."

Today, the volunteers are identified by their red jackets and can be seen anywhere in the hospital. They may be seen helping in the Emergency Department, particularly spending time with children whose siblings are being attended by a physician or a nurse, comforting parents, spending time in the DAT area, offering child care in Emily's Backyard or in the well-known cuddlers program. In this program, volunteers come in and cuddle babies whose parents live out of town or are unable to visit

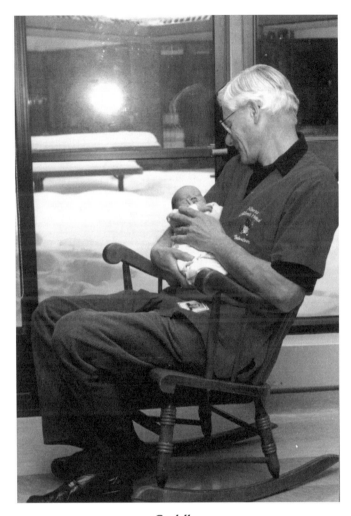

Cuddler.

frequently. There are many other volunteer activities which are not so obvious, but are essential to the smooth running of the hospital.

The activities of the volunteers attest to the strong connection between the Alberta Children's Hospital and the community of Calgary and southern Alberta.❖

References

1. *The Calgary Herald*, March 13, 1965.
2. Lil McAra, personal communication.
3. *Minutes*. Alberta Children's Hospital Board, November 6, 1959.
4. *Annual Report*. Alberta Children's Hospital, 1966.

PART EIGHT

A LOOK
TO THE FUTURE

❖❖❖❖❖❖❖❖❖❖❖❖❖❖

O ur book started with a description of Calgary early this century
   and will end with projections for the future.
      The Calgary Regional Health Authority (CRHA) now has re-
sponsibility for all aspects of child health. The Alberta Children's Hospital has a new, and potentially exciting, role as the main site of child
health care, now operating as a hub connected to different spokes. The
Alberta Children's Hospital can be regarded as the hub, while the many
other aspects of health-care services for children are the spokes. Examples of spokes are paediatric outreach clinics, paediatric emergency care
and in-patient areas in other hospitals. The hub and the spokes are inti-
mately connected, and services should be accessible according to the
needs of the child. Children should now be able to move from one segment of the service to another without barriers. The Alberta Children's
Hospital will serve to assist the "spokes" in the management of selected
patients, while on other occasions referring children to an outside agency,
recognizing that we are all part of a larger community.

Child health professionals are firmly committed to preventing childhood afflictions. This means that while specific efforts to improve hygiene and advocate immunization will continue, new ones must be
developed to address issues such as the prevention of injuries. The role
of environmental factors in causing childhood disease and the identifica-
tion of conditions during pregnancy that may lead to prematurity, congenital malformations or disorders that may affect the newborn child will
receive close attention. Some neonatal illnesses become chronic and cause
long-term challenges to children and their families. However, within the
paediatric organization, the child will remain in the centre.

The Alberta Children's Hospital will continue to be the site for more
specialized and intensive care and the delivery of high-technology inter-
ventions. There are many examples including minimally invasive surgery,
bone-marrow transplants, gene therapy and the use of techniques to correct cardiac anomalies without surgery.

The Alberta Children's Hospital will also explore new avenues in the
active involvement of children and parents in planning and developing

health care so that children can continue to receive the best possible care, right here in southern Alberta. There is a long history of involving parents in the care of their own children and also in the management of the hospital. This involvement is so firmly entrenched that parents are well represented on committees planning improvements in child health care. This parental involvement will continue and may increase.

We hope that the new health-care structure will benefit children and adolescents, but there are potential dangers of regionalization. For example, will the ultimate decision-makers, with many responsibilities, still protect the interests of children, a small group statistically? There is a danger that adult standards will be applied across CRHA, without considering the specific, and often time-consuming, medical needs of children. A trivial example that illustrates the whole problem is drawing blood from children. Those working with children know that it takes much longer to draw blood from a child than from an adult and also requires two professionals rather than one. Will such examples be recognized by managers who have a large responsibility and strict budget requirements to meet? These ultimate decision-makers may not be part of the Alberta Children's Hospital or even knowledgeable about paediatric issues. They are likely concerned and preoccupied with the problems of the increasing number of older people in society.

Under regionalization, the Alberta Children's Hospital itself no longer has a unified administration. Many of the services which were not seen as "clinical services" came under different branches of the centralized administration. These varied from services with an obvious clinical relevance such as audiovisual services, library and volunteer services to areas with less obvious clinical relevance, such as finance, maintenance and other support services. All of these areas include individuals with knowledge of the special needs of children and a children's hospital, who have a high level of commitment to children and to ACH. Their knowledge and commitment could easily be lost.

Even if the process of regionalization goes well, there are still dangers from decentralization of delivery of care. If there are too many outreach services, it may be difficult for paediatric professionals to interact with one another, so special attention must be given to this aspect.

All children in southern Alberta, no matter how small the community they live in, must have access to the best medical care. This means that local emergency departments must have suitable arrangements in place for children. Advances in communication, such as satellite conferences, provide many creative possibilities to deal with challenging situations. Paediatric health-care professionals will continue to collaborate to improve care for all children and also to ensure that the needs of children are identified by those in authority. Parents and professionals will also continue their collaboration.❖

ALBERTA CHILDREN'S HOSPITAL NAMES

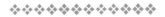

1922-49	Junior Red Cross Children's Hospital
1949-51	Red Cross Crippled Children's Hospital
1951-58	Alberta Red Cross Crippled Children's Hospital
1958-59	Alberta Crippled Children's Hospital
1959-81	Alberta Children's Hospital
1981-present	Alberta Children's Hospital Child Health Centre

(From 1972 to present also known as Alberta Children's Provincial General Hospital)

DIRECTORS OF NURSING[1]

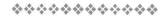

1922-26	Miss Peat
1926-27	Miss Elliott
1927-??	Miss Lynn
19??-32	Miss Arnold
1932-33	Miss Davidson
1933-52	Florence Reid
1952-65	Margaret Baxter
1965-80	Dorothy Potts
1980-81	Barbara Racine
1981-84	Andree De Filippi[2]
1984-90	Nora Greenley[2,3]
1988-93	Moira Cameron (Joint)
1988-93	Diane Ellingson (Joint)
1993-present	Diane Ellingson[4]

1   The title of Director of Nursing did not exist after 1993.
2   Administrator, In-patient Division
3   Vice-President, Patient Care Services, in the spring of 1990, and Senior Operating Officer, Child Health Services, in 1994.
4   Director, Patient Care Services, in 1993 and Interim Administrative Leader, Child Health Services, in 1994, was appointed Administrative Leader, Child Health Services, in 1997.

APPENDIX THREE

ADMINISTRATORS
ALBERTA CHILDREN'S HOSPITAL[1]

❖❖❖❖❖❖❖❖❖❖❖❖❖

1922-57	Commissioner, Alberta Division, Canadian Red Cross
1958-71	S.V. Pryce
1971-89	R. Innes (Executive Director)
1989-95	J. Saunders (President)

1 After 1995, under Calgary Regional Authority administration

APPENDIX FOUR

ADMINISTRATORS
ALBERTA CHILDREN'S HOSPITAL
FOUNDATION

❖❖❖❖❖❖❖❖❖❖❖❖❖

1973-79	Basil Hill
1978-79	A.P. Taylor
1979-84	Hugh C. Boucher
1984-93	Julius Lister
1993-95	Frank Rosar (Executive Director).
1996-present	Maureen Sheahan (Executive Director).

APPENDIX FIVE

BOARD CHAIR
ALBERTA CHILDREN'S
HOSPITAL[1]

❖❖❖❖❖❖❖❖❖❖❖❖❖

1958-72	Mervyn G. Graves
1972-81	K. Manning
1981-85	F.W. Fitzpatrick
1985-87	J. Maybin
1987-90	J. Davidson
1990-94	J. Herbison

1 Position abolished with regionalization

BOARD CHAIR
ALBERTA CHILDREN'S HOSPITAL
FOUNDATION

❖❖❖❖❖❖❖❖❖❖❖❖❖

1972-85	Mervyn G. Graves
1986-88	William H. Tye
1989-89	Flora Allison
1989-91	John Fisher
1991-93	Herb Stoll
1993-94	Bob Millar
1995-96	Allen Hagerman
1996-present	Charles Fischer

INDEX

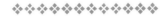

ABOUT THE AUTHORS

❖❖❖❖❖❖❖❖❖❖❖❖❖❖

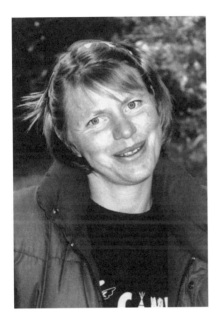

Arty Coppes-Zantinga was born in the Netherlands and obtained her Masters of Arts from the University of Leiden in 1981. She came to Calgary in 1993.

She has been writing articles on the history of medicine since 1992 and in 1996 became Special Features Editor of the *Journal of Medical and Paediatric Oncology*.

She has an adjunct appointment in the Department of Oncology, Faculty of Medicine at The University of Calgary and is a historical consultant at Alberta Children's Hospital.

Arty lives in Calgary with her husband and three young children.

❖❖❖❖❖❖❖❖❖❖❖❖❖❖

Ian Mitchell was born in Scotland and graduated in Medicine from the University of Edinburgh in 1968. He trained in paediatrics in Scotland and Canada and has been on the staff at the Alberta Children's Hospital since 1982.

He is a Professor of Paediatrics at The University of Calgary and has a general interest in health care issues affecting children. His interest in the history of paediatrics led to the formation of a group to preserve records and artifacts at Alberta Children's Hospital.

Ian is a Canadian citizen and lives in Calgary with his wife. He has two grown-up sons.

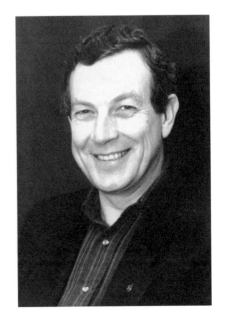